Diabetes & Cardiovascular Disease

A Practical Primer

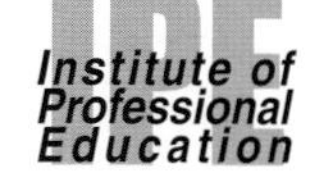

LSU HEALTH SCIENCES CENTER

Louisiana State University School of Medicine
New Orleans, Louisiana

Institute of Professional Education
LSU Health Sciences Center
1600 Canal Street, Suite 1034
New Orleans, Louisiana 70112

ISBN 0-9704788-0-1

Preface

The clinician who treats patients with cardiovascular diseases commonly encounters diabetes mellitus as a co-morbid condition. Additionally, diabetic patients with cardiovascular diseases also have other co-morbidities, most commonly hypertension, renal disease and lipid abnormalities. Thus, the clinician is challenged with devising a treatment plan that incorporates the therapeutic goals associated with all of the patient's conditions. It is this challenge that stimulated the writing of this primer.

A distinguished group of clinician-scientists have contributed their expertise to the preparation of this book. The various chapters deal with the more commonly encountered clinical problems that arise in the care of the diabetic patient with cardiovascular disease: the lifestyle and pharmacologic strategies for glycemic management, the detection and evaluation of significant coronary atherosclerosis, the ever-present hypertension and the necessity for rigorous blood pressure control, the treatment of heart failure, the prevention of renal disease, the diagnosis of peripheral arterial disease, the management of dyslipidemias and special considerations regarding the selection of agents to control blood glucose.

The authors have tried, where possible, to provide advice supported by clinical trial evidence. We are well aware that other experts may have differing approaches to the clinical problems addressed in this primer. However, we feel that this primer will serve as a reliable foundation for approaching the difficult problems of caring for the diabetic patient with cardiovascular disease. And lastly, we believe that this primer will contribute to the ability of the clinician to deliver comprehensive, non-fragmented care for the patient with the result of better outcomes.

Disclaimer

The opinions expressed in this publication are those of the authors and do not necessarily reflect the opinions or recommendations of their affiliated institutions, the Institute of Professional Education, Louisiana State University Health Sciences Center, Louisiana State University, the publisher, SmithKline Beecham, Inc., or any other persons. Any procedures, medications or other courses of diagnosis or treatment discussed or suggested by the authors should not be used by clinicians without evaluation of their patients' conditions and of possible contraindications or dangers in use, review of any applicable manufacturers' recommendations, and comparison with the recommendations of authorities.

Acknowledgments

I would be remiss if I didn't thank the staff of the Institute of Professional Education and the Cardiovascular Research Section for all their help in bringing this project to reality. I also want to thank SmithKline Beecham for their unrestricted educational subsidy that made this project possible. TDG

Editor in Chief

Thomas D. Giles, MD
Professor of Medicine
Director, Cardiovascular Research
LSU School of Medicine
New Orleans, LA

Co-editors

James R. Sowers, MD
Professor of Medicine and Cell Biology
Director, Endocrinology, Diabetes and Hypertension
SUNY Health Sciences Center at Brooklyn
Brooklyn, NY

Michael A. Weber, MD
Associate Dean for Clinical Investigation
Professor of Medicine
SUNY Downstate College of Medicine
Brooklyn, NY

Contributing Authors

George L. Bakris, MD
Director, Hypertension Research
Rush Presbyterian St. Luke's Medical Center
Chicago, IL

Peter A. Brady, MD
Instructor in Medicine
Mayo Medical School
Rochester, MN

Alan Chait, MD
Professor of Medicine
University of Washington School of Medicine
Seattle, WA

Stephen M. Factor, MD
Chairman, Surgical Pathology
Jacobi Medical Center/ North Central Bronx Hospital
Professor of Pathology
Professor of Medicine (Cardiology)
Albert Einstein College of Medicine
Bronx, NY

Merri L. Pendergrass, MD
Assistant Professor of Medicine
Tulane University School of Medicine
New Orleans, LA

Gary E. Sander, MD, PhD
Professor of Medicine
LSU School of Medicine
New Orleans, LA

Other Contributors

Tami Hotard, MA
Editorial Consultant
LSU School of Medicine
New Orleans, LA

Mica Foret, BA
Graphic Designer/Medical Editor
Institute of Professional Education
LSU Heatlh Sciences Center
New Orleans, LA

Table of Contents

The Cardiovascular Pathology of Diabetes Mellitus

Stephen M. Factor, MD

Introduction

Diabetes mellitus is a systemic disease with pathological effects on tissues and organs throughout the body. Pathological changes result from diabetes-induced metabolic perturbations (e.g. fatty liver) and complications of infection (e.g. pyelonephritis), damage that leads to significant morbidity and mortality results from cardiovascular disease. Virtually all of the major complications of diabetes mellitus are mediated through disease of blood vessels: ischemic heart disease and peripheral vascular disease (large vessels); stroke (large and small vessels); cardiomyopathy (small vessels and microvasculature); arterionephrosclerosis (small vessels); retinopathy (microvasculature); and, nodular glomerulosclerosis or Kimmelstiel-Wilson disease (microvasculature). In most cases, there is an interaction between blood vessels of all calibers leading to tissue and organ damage. In addition, hypertension, which is markedly increased in prevalence in diabetes mellitus, exacerbates vascular disease and contributes to tissue pathology. Thus, a recognition of the vascular abnormalities in diabetes mellitus is critical to understanding the pathology of the syndrome. This chapter will discuss the macrovascular and microvascular complications, and because of its significant role in the morbidity and mortality in diabetic patients, will focus on the myocardium. Further, the role of hypertension and its interaction with the vascular alterations to modify and increase tissue injury will be addressed.

Definitions

Before we can discuss vascular disease, it is necessary to define what is meant by macrovasculature, small muscular vessels and microvasculature. In general, because diabetic pathology is primarily limited to the arterial side of the circulation, these terms refer to arteries and their branches down to the capillaries. The macrovasculature consists of the aorta (an elastic artery) and its muscular branches to 1000 μm in diameter. Thus, the coronary arteries, the carotid arteries, and the femoral arteries would be components of the macrovasculature. Small muscular arteries (or small vessels) consist of vessels ranging from 1000 μm to vessels 100 to 200 μm in size. The prominent intramyocardial arteries that course through the myocardium fall into this category. The microvasculature consists of arterioles and capillaries. Renal glomerular vessels and the vessels directly supplying nutrients to individual myocytes are examples of the microvasculature that is affected pathologically in diabetes mellitus.

Macrovasculature

Despite the fact that so many of the major complications of diabetes mellitus are the result of macrovascular disease, there is nothing specific that identifies the vascular pathology as diabetic in origin. Diabetes has been recognized as a contributing risk factor for atherosclerosis for more than 50 years. Since hypertension and serum lipid abnormalities are common in diabetics, it is difficult to separate the effects of these abnormalities from the diabetic state. It is noteworthy that diabetic animals without hypertension and without hypercholesterolemia do not develop atherosclerotic plaques in the macrovasculature. The atherosclerotic plaques in the diabetic patient are not unique.

Atherosclerosis tends to occur at an earlier age in diabetic patients when compared to age and gender matched controls, and it tends to be more severe and widespread throughout the vascular tree. It is also unpredictable. It is not at all uncommon, for example, to see patients with diabetes for greater than 10 years with extensive aortic and peripheral vascular disease, but minimal carotid and coronary artery lesions. Similarly, patients may have severe occlusive coronary disease and multiple myocardial infarctions, with minimal involvement of the aorta. Since diabetics get more severe atherosclerosis at an earlier age than non-diabetics, diabetes mellitus is considered to be a cause of accelerated atherosclerosis. All of the complications of atherosclerosis are more prevalent in diabetics, and more severe (see Table 1.1 and Fig. 1.1).

The presence of complex atherosclerotic plaques (with extensive lipid, connective tissue matrix and calcium) makes the diabetic patient susceptible to tissue ischemia, thrombosis and tissue infarction, and atheroemboli. Involvement of the aorta may lead to aneurysm formation and potential rupture. Ischemia and eventual gangrene of the lower extremities may be initiated with ilio-femoral artery occlusion (atherosclerotic, or thrombotic, or both), and occlusive disease of the major arteries down to the foot (popliteal, anterior and posterior tibial).

Table 1.1

Atherosclerotic complications in diabetes mellitus
1. Tissue Ischemia
a. Infarction (Myocardial, Cerebral, Renal)
b. Angina Pectoris
c. Cerebrovascular Insufficiency (Transient Ischemic Attacks)
d. Peripheral Vascular Disease (Claudication)
e. Peripheral Vascular Disease (Ulceration, Infection, Gangrene)
2. Aortic Aneurysm, with and without rupture
3. Vascular Thrombosis and Embolism
4. Atheroembolism (Cholesterol Emboli)

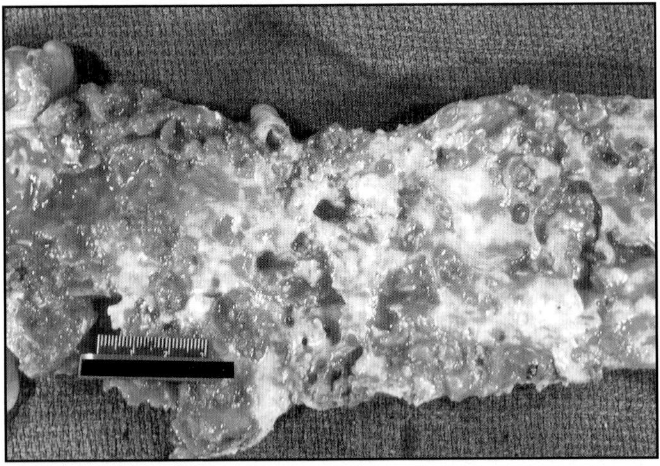

Figure 1.1. Severely atherosclerotic abdominal aorta from a diabetic patient. There are multiple ulcerating and thrombosed plaques affecting the entire intimal surface and the branch vessels. Although not specific for diabetes, this degree of severe atherosclerosis is common.

It is of interest that there is an increased prevalence of non-atherosclerotic disease of the lower extremity macrovasculature that contributes to vascular insufficiency, claudication, and gangrene. Specifically, Monckeberg's medial sclerosis, which begins as calcification of the internal elastic lamina, and then may spread to involve the media and intima with calcium and connective tissue deposition and lead to luminal thrombosis, is often observed in amputation specimens (Fig. 1.2). Monckeberg's medial sclerosis is of unknown cause, and is not only seen in diabetic peripheral vascular disease.

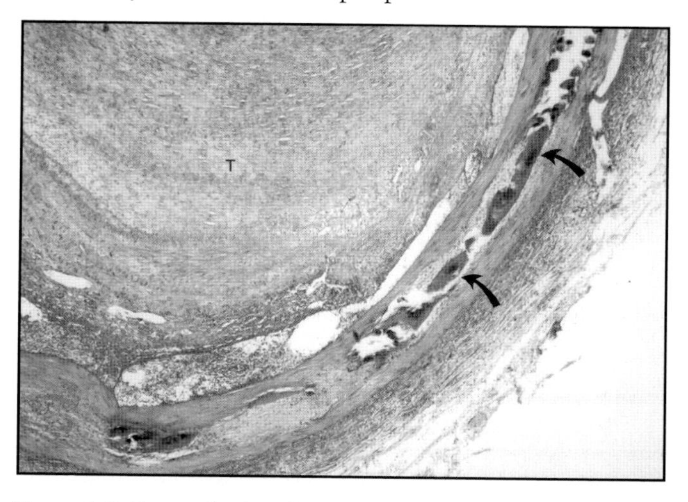

Figure 1.2. Femoral artery from an ischemic leg of a patient with diabetes mellitus affected by Monckeberg's medial sclerosis and calcification. The lumen was remotely thrombosed (T). The medial smooth muscle has almost circumferential calcifications (arrows) that begin in the internal elastic membrane and then spread into the intima and medial layers. This condition is common in diabetics, and it is independent of atherosclerosis. (H & E stain, original magnification 12.5X).

The role of the macrovasculature in myocardial pathology is generally well-understood. Diabetic patients are apt to develop myocardial infarctions which are often larger and more likely to be transmural than would be expected when compared to non-diabetics with similar infarctions. Diabetic myocardial infarctions are often clinically silent (up to 25 to 30 percent, or higher). Infarction of the myocardium is less well-tolerated by diabetic patients than in non-diabetics with similarly sized infarctions, and it may lead to significant ventricular failure and death. Poor clinical outcomes following an infarction may be the result of chronic cardiomyopathic damage to the myocardium secondary to microvascular disease, which makes the myocardium more susceptible to coronary artery ischemia.

It is not uncommon for patients to have multi-focal areas of myocardial necrosis in different stages of development and healing (Fig. 1.3, 1.4). These areas of necrosis are often macroscopic, and they may extend across the ventricular wall. However, rather than being the result of a single event (e.g. acute coronary thrombosis), they represent multiple episodes of coronary-induced ischemia, which may show organization and healing consistent with several weeks duration. They are the equivalent of a myocardial infarction, but they are actually indicative of progressive, intermittent ischemia. Clinically, they may be diagnosed as a myocardial infarction, or progressive ventricular failure.

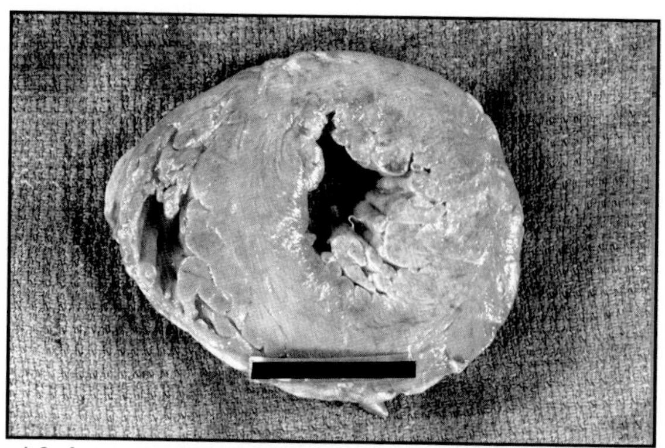

Figure 1.3. A cross-section of the left and right ventricular walls from a patient with hypertensive and diabetic cardiomyopathy. Note the marked left ventricular mural hypertrophy with a small left ventricular cavity. Also, observe the mottled pale and dark discoloration of the ventricular wall characteristic of multiple stages of necrosis and fibrosis.

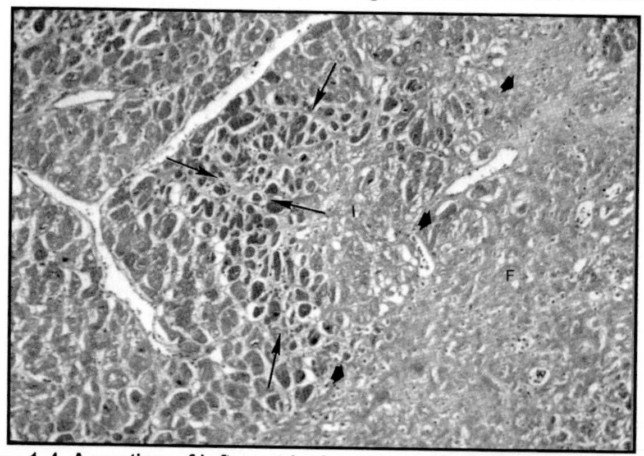

Figure 1.4. A section of left ventricular myocardium from a patient with hypertensive and diabetic cardiomyopathy. There are multiple stages of necrosis and healing. Note the fibrosis (F) demarcated by arrow heads, in which the ghost outlines of previously necrosed myocytes are visible, characteristic of reperfusion necrosis. Adjacent to this zone, there is a region of ischemic damage (I), and then a small area of acute reperfusion necrosis (arrows). The myocardium surrounding this area also has chronic ischemic damage. (H & E stain, original magnification 31X).

Microvasculature

Small vessel disease is commonly observed in the diabetic heart, as well as systemically. Lesions consist of concentric small muscle hypertrophy and hyperplasia associated with connective tissue, and variable degrees of intimal thickening (Fig. 1.5). Such changes are also termed vascular sclerosis (or hardening). They are not unique features of diabetes, as similar changes may occur secondary to hypertension, which may account for the majority of such changes in diabetics who are also hypertensive. In the heart, the vascular sclerosis is often associated with perivascular fibrosis, which may extend between myocardial fibers as interstitial fibrosis.

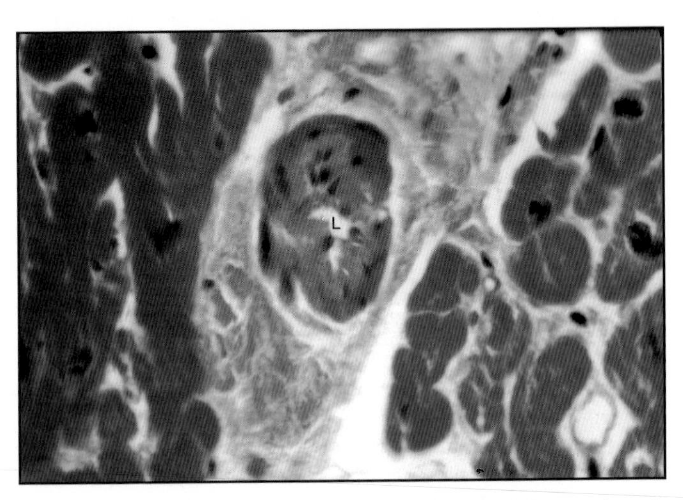

Figure 1.5. A small intramyocardial artery with severe sclerosis and a markedly narrowed lumen (L). The vessel has perivascular fibrosis. (Masson's trichrome stain, original magnification 80X).

Thus, there may be a contribution to the fine scarring in the myocardium characteristic of diabetic cardiomyopathy. However, though small vessel disease is relatively common in diabetic hearts, attempts to quantify its frequency, and to relate its presence to the development of significant myocardial damage, have not been particularly rewarding. This lack of correlation between vascular sclerosis and other parameters of myocardial pathology also has been confirmed by experimental studies. Since the small muscular arteries in the heart are resistance vessels, it is possible that their hypertrophy and thickening is in response to more distal vascular pathology.

The microcirculation in the diabetic heart is abnormal, and it may contribute significantly to myocardial pathology leading to diabetic cardiomyopathy. It has been known for many years that diabetic capillaries have thickened basal lamina, hypothesized to limit oxygen and nutrient transport across the vessel wall, thereby leading to metabolic myocellular dysfunction and ischemia. It also has been suggested that the diabetic microvasculature is abnormally "leaky," and so may contribute to interstitial edema and inflammation, which may stimulate interstitial connective tissue synthesis. Over two decades ago, we used silicone rubber perfusions of diabetic hearts at post-mortem, and we demonstrated the presence of arteriolar and capillary microaneurysms, similar to those seen in the retina (Fig. 1.6). Subsequently, microaneurysms of the glomerular capillary loops have been described, and recognized as

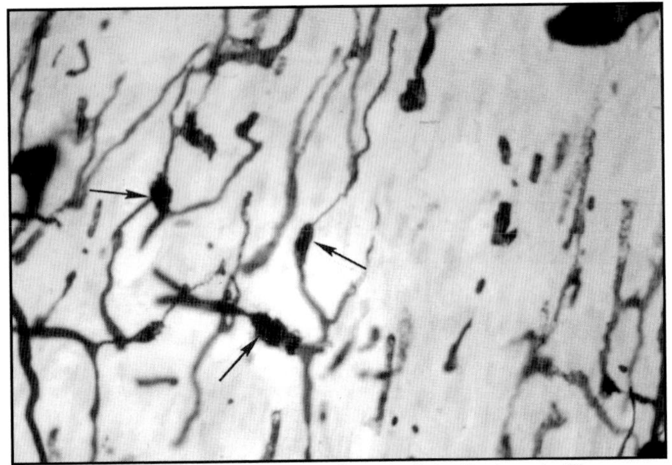

Figure 1.6. Silicone rubber perfused diabetic heart. There are multiple aneurysms in the microcirculation (arrows), similar to microaneurysms in the diabetic retina and renal glomerulus. (Unstained, cleared myocardium, original magnification 80X).

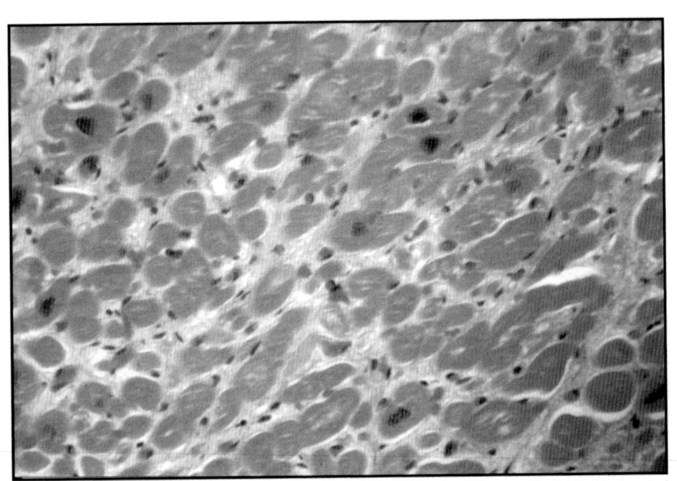

Figure 1.7. Left ventricular myocardium from a hypertensive and diabetic patient with cardiomyopathy. There is myocellular hypertrophy, and diffuse interstitial fibrosis. (H & E stain, original magnification 80X).

the precursor to the glomerular nodule of Kimmelstiel-Wilson disease (the only pathognomonic lesion in diabetic vascular disease) suggesting that arteriolar and capillary microaneurysms are a systemic phenomenon in diabetes mellitus, albeit one that requires either special vascular beds (e.g. retina and glomerulus), or special techniques (e.g. silicone rubber perfusion) to demonstrate it. Whether the microaneurysm, per se, is the cause of tissue injury or is secondary to pathogenetic mechanisms that also lead to myocardial injury could not be determined from clinical studies. Specifically, microvascular spasm may lead to damage of the microvascular wall and subsequent microaneurysm formation, and, may also lead to reperfusion injury to the myocardial tissue.

Diabetic Cardiomyopathy

Multifocal areas of myocardial fibrosis (interstitial, replacement, and perivascular), together with small vessel sclerosis, and myocellular hypertrophy, often occurring in the absence of significant occlusive coronary artery disease, defines diabetic cardiomyopathy (Fig. 1.7). Such hearts are generally markedly hypertrophied (450-600 gms), with left and right ventricular wall thickening, and relatively small ventricular cavities, but often dilated atrial chambers. The hearts in diabetic cardiomyopathy are stiff hearts, and if patients manifest congestive heart failure, it is often diastolic in origin. Although systolic dysfunction also may occur and the left ventricular wall may thin and the cavity dilate, particularly if there is coronary artery atherosclerosis and macrovascular-induced ischemia, diastolic dysfunction is more common. The pathology is bi-ventricular with scarring often present in the right ventricle suggesting that the pathogenesis of the myocardial damage is mediated through systemic circulating factors, such as hormones or cytokines that act at the myocellular or vascular level.

Hypertension

As noted previously, hypertension is very prevalent in patients with chronic diabetes (up to 75 percent of those diabetic for more than 10 years), and it contributes to the retinopathy, nephropathy, and atherosclerotic complications of the disease. Similarly, hypertension appears to have a significant pathogenetic role in the development of diabetic cardiomyopathy. Studies of human hearts at autopsy, from groups that were diabetic and normotensive, diabetic and hypertensive, and hypertensive alone, demonstrated marked increases in heart weight and myocardial fibrosis when diabetes occurred together with hypertension.

Conclusions

As summarized in this chapter, diabetic pathology is generalized, but much of the tissue damage results from abnormal blood vessels of all sizes. Thus, ischemia and infarction is predominantly a macrovascular disease due to atherosclerosis; whereas, retinopathy, nephropathy, and cardiomyopathy are predominantly microvascular diseases due to structural and functional abnormalities of the microcirculation. The metabolic perturbations of diabetes undoubtedly play a role in tissue and organ damage (e.g. glycosylation of hemoglobin leading to decreased oxygen release from red blood cells, and non-enzymatic glycosylation of connective tissue which may affect oxygen and nutrient transport from capillaries to cells). Hypertension acts together with diabetes to exacerbate pathology. However, the common pathway of the pathology is generally mediated through the macrovasculature and the microvasculature.

Selected References:

1. Stearns S, Schlesinger MJ, Rudy A: Incidence and clinical significance of coronary artery disease in diabetes mellitus. Arch Int Med 1947, 80:463-474.
2. Bryfogle JW, Bradley RF: The vascular complications of diabetes mellitus: a clinical study. Diabetes 1957, 6:159-167.
3. Kannel WB, McGee DL: Diabetes and cardiovascular disease: the Framingham study. JAMA 1979, 241: 2035-2038.
4. Factor SM, Minase T, Sonnenblick EH: Clinical and morphological features of human hypertensive-diabetic cardiomyopathy. Am Heart J 1980, 99:446-458.
5. Factor SM, Okun EM, Minase T: Capillary microaneurysms in the human diabetic heart. N Engl J Med 1980, 302:384-388.
6. Lemp GF, Vander Zwaag R, Hughes JP, et al.: Association between the severity of diabetes mellitus and coronary arterial atherosclerosis. Am J Cardiol 1987, 60:1015-1019.
7. van Hoeven KH, Factor SM: Diabetic heart disease: the clinical and pathological spectrum. Part I and Part II. Clin Cardiol 1989, 12:600-604; 667-671.

8. van Hoeven KH, Factor SM: A comparison of the pathological spectrum of hypertensive, diabetic, and hypertensive-diabetic heart disease. Circulation 1990, 82:848-855.

9. Factor SM, Borczuk A, Charron MJ, Fein FS, van Hoeven KH, Sonnenblick EH: Myocardial alterations in diabetes and hypertension. Diabetes Res Clin Pract 1996, 31: Suppl S133-S142.

Pathophysiology and Management of Type 2 Diabetes

Merri L. Pendergrass, MD, PhD

Introduction

Treatment of type 2 diabetes is becoming increasingly challenging. Insulin and five classes of oral therapies currently are available for treating hyperglycemia. Additional classes are under development and likely will become available in the near future. All of the available oral therapies can be effective at lowering the blood glucose level in appropriately selected patients. The different classes, however, have different mechanisms of action and metabolic effects (Table 2.1), safety concerns (Table 2.2), and dosing and cost considerations (Tables 2.3, 2.4). These issues, as well as strategies for combining oral agents and insulin, will be discussed in this chapter. The various treatment modalities for hyperglycemia also may affect cardiovascular function via effects on non-traditional cardiovascular risk factors, endothelial function, vascular resistance, and other factors that are not yet well-understood. These effects are beyond the scope of this chapter and will not be discussed.

Therapeutic Goals

Because hyperglycemia plays an important role in the pathogenesis of microvascular (retinopathy, neuropathy, nephropathy), and probably macrovascular (cardiovascular, cerebrovascular, peripheral vascular) complications of diabetes, blood glucose levels should be reduced to as near to normal as possible. The American Diabetes Association recommends a treatment goal of a fasting plasma glucose (FPG) less than 120 mg/dl and an HbA_{1c} level of less than 7%. Further actions, i.e., medication adjustment and behavior modification, are indicated when the FPG level is less than 80 mg/dl or greater than 140 mg/dl, or the HbA_{1c} level exceeds 8%. Type 2 diabetes often occurs as part of a complex cluster of metabolic disorders (the Insulin Resistance Syndrome, Metabolic Syndrome or Syndrome X) that includes obesity, hypertension, dyslipidemia, clotting abnormalities, microalbuminuria, and accelerated atherosclerosis. Because coronary heart disease represents the major cause of death in type 2 diabetes, cardiovascular risk factors must be aggressively treated (see chapters IV and V). Moreover, it is desirable that any anti-hyperglycemic agent has favorable effects, or has minimal adverse effects, on known cardiovascular risk factors.

Pathogenesis of Type 2 Diabetes

The appropriate treatment of type 2 diabetes is based on an understanding of its pathophysiology. Type 2 diabetes is a heterogeneous and multifactorial disease characterized by defects in both insulin action (insulin resistance) and insulin secretion. The relative contribution of each of these abnormalities varies both between patients and during the course of the disease in an individual patient.

Insulin resistance usually is present in the earliest stages of type 2 diabetes, as well as in normal-glucose tolerant individuals who are at risk of developing the disease ("prediabetes"). It is manifest in the liver as excessive glucose production, particularly in the basal state. The increased rate of basal hepatic glucose production is closely related to an elevated fasting plasma glucose level, which is the major determinant of the mean day-long blood glucose level. Insulin resistance in the muscle is manifest as decreased glucose uptake in response to a meal. This, along with excessive hepatic glucose production, contributes to the excessive post-prandial increase in plasma glucose level in diabetic patients. It follows that agents that reduce insulin resistance in the liver and muscle will be effective at improving the glycemic control. Agents that reduce insulin resistance are referred to as "insulin sensitizers." Since insulin resistance is reported to be an independent risk factor for coronary heart disease, insulin sensitizers may have unique cardioprotective benefits, in addition to glucose-lowering effects. This theory remains unproven in clinical research.

Impaired insulin secretion also plays a major role in the pathogenesis of type 2 diabetes. Type 2 diabetes is characterized by both a *delay* and a *decrease* in meal-stimulated insulin secretion. The delay in insulin secretion contributes to the excessive early post-prandial rise in blood glucose levels. The decrease in insulin secretion may be reflected by a *relative*, rather than an *absolute* insulin deficiency. Plasma insulin concentrations are usually increased in non-diabetic individuals at risk for diabetes. This is thought to reflect compensation by the pancreas to overcome insulin resistance. As long as the pancreas is able to sustain high levels of insulin secretion, glucose tolerance remains normal. In the natural history of type 2 diabetes, for reasons that remain unclear, the ability of the pancreas to secrete insulin progressively declines (Fig. 2.1). Insulin levels in early diabetes may be elevated, in absolute terms. However, relative to the severity of insulin resistance and prevailing hyperglycemia, even these elevated plasma insulin levels are not sufficient to maintain euglycemia. Once the overt hyperglycemia has developed, the decline in glycemic control is relentless. In later stages of diabetes, insulin levels may become deficient in absolute terms, which results in severely elevated plasma glucose levels.

Figure 2.1

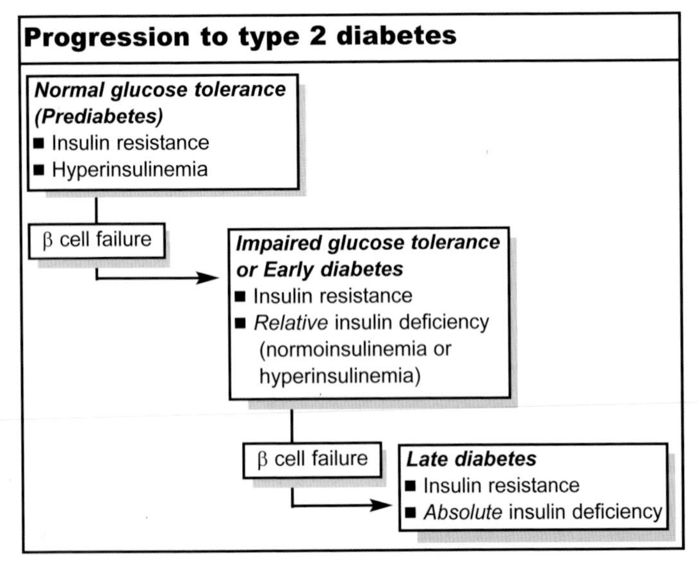

From the above discussion it follows that drugs that improve insulin secretion may be effective in treating type 2 diabetes.

Treatment Strategy

As discussed above, hyperglycemia in patients with type 2 diabetes results from an imbalance between insulin secretion and insulin resistance. Thus, during the hyperinsulinemic or normoinsulinemic phases of diabetes, nonpharmacological strategies that reduce insulin secretory requirements (diet) or increase insulin effectiveness (exercise and weight loss) may be effective at lowering the blood glucose. When these behavioral measures fail to achieve the desired level of glycemic control, pharmacologic intervention is necessary. The currently available pharmacological agents work by three mechanisms: enhancing insulin secretion, improving insulin action, or decreasing carbohydrate absorption.

Figure 2.2

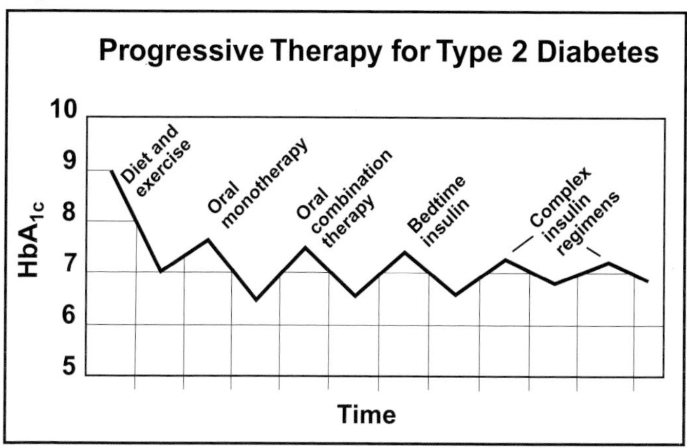

Furthermore, therapy for hyperglycemia in patients with type 2 diabetes may be focused specifically on decreasing *fasting glucose*, and/or *postprandial glucose.* In most patients with type 2 diabetes, insulin secretory ability decreases with time. This important observation emphasizes the need for constant reassessment of the diabetic patient and appropriate adjustment of the therapeutic regimen in order to maintain the desired level of glycemic control. Even patients with good initial response to therapy usually will eventually require a second or third medication. Effective treatment generally will require the combined use of diet, exercise, oral agents and eventually insulin (Fig. 2.2).

Oral Agents

Drugs That Enhance Insulin Secretion

Sulfonylureas

Sufonylureas have been the mainstay of antidiabetic therapy for >40 years. The controversial University Group Diabetes Program study, published in 1970, first raised concerns that sulfonylureas may increase the risk of cardiovascular death. Results from the United Kingdom Prospective Diabetes Study, published in 1998, have largely assuaged these concerns, although this issue continues to be investigated (see chapter VIII). In that study sulfonylureas were not found to have an adverse effect on cardiovascular outcomes.

The primary mechanism of action of sulfonylureas is enhancement of insulin secretion by the pancreas (Fig. 2.3).

The hypoglycemic potential of sulfonylureas is directly related to the starting plasma glucose level. The higher the FPG, the greater the decrease from baseline. In the U.S. the mean HbA_{1c} value in diabetic patients is ~10%, corresponding to a FPG level of >200 mg/dl. In such patients, the expected effect of sulfonylureas is a decrease in the FPG of 60-70 mg/dl and in the HbA_{1c}

Figure 2.3

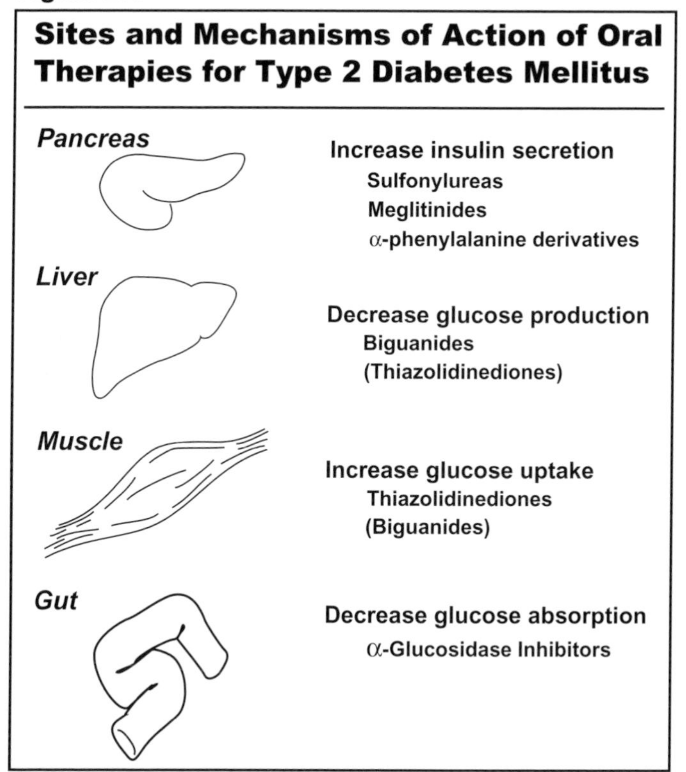

by 1.5-2.0%. First generation sulfonylureas (chlorpropamide, tolazamide, tolbutamide, and acetohexamide) are now rarely used because of excessive side

Table 2.1

Comparison of oral antidiabetic medications used as monotherapy

	Increase insulin secretion		Improve insulin action		Modify intestinal absorption
Class	***Sulfonylureas***	***Meglitinides***	***Biguanides***	***Thiazolidine-diones***	***Alpha glucosidase inhibitors***
Agents	Glipizide, Glyburide, Glimepiride	Repaglinide	Metformin	Rosiglitazone, Pioglitazone	Acarbose, Miglitol
Primary site of action	Pancreas	Pancreas	Liver	Muscle	Gut
Primary mechanism of action	Increase insulin secretion	Increase insulin secretion	Decrease hepatic glucose production	Increase glucose uptake	Delay carbohydrate absorption
Approximate FPG lowering (mg/dl)	60-70	60-70	60-70	35-40	20-30
Approximate HbA_{1c} lowering (%)	1.5-2.0	1.5-2.0	1.5-2.0	1.0-1.2	0.5-1.0
Effect on plasma insulin	↑	↑	↓	↓	↓ ↔
Effect on body weight	↑	↑	↓	↑	↔
Effect on total cholesterol	↔	↔	↓	↑	↔
Effect on LDL	↔	↔	↓	↑	↔
Effect on HDL	↔	↔	↔	↑	↔
Effect on TG	↔	↔	↓	↓	↔

effects and drug interactions. The second-generation sulfonylureas, glyburide, glipizide and glimepiride, are all equally effective in lowering glucose.

In most studies, sulfonylureas have been reported to have generally neutral effects on plasma lipids. Sulfonylurea therapy commonly is associated with a mild weight gain (Table 2.1).

Table 2.2

Comparison of adverse effects and safety issues in oral antidiabetic medications

	Primary precautions and contraindications	*Monitoring parameters*	*Hypo-glycemia*	*Most common adverse effects*
Sulfonylureas	▪ Predisposition to severe hypoglycemia, e.g. severe liver or kidney disease		Yes	Hypoglycemia
Meglitinides	▪ Predisposition to severe hypoglycemia, e.g. severe liver or kidney disease		Yes	Hypoglycemia
Biguanides	▪ Creatinine > 1.5 males or > 1.4 females ▪ CHF requiring drug treatment ▪ Excessive alcohol use, significant liver disease, severe infection, respiratory insufficiency, hypox-emia ▪ Hold after contrast studies	– Baseline and annual creatinine periodic liver function tests. – Baseline and periodic hemato-logic parameters.	No	Abdominal discomfort Diarrhea
Thiazolidine-diones ("Glitazones")	▪ Abnormal liver function tests ▪ CHF NYHA Class III or IV	Liver function tests: q2 months x 1 yr, then periodically	No	Edema, anemia
Alpha Glucosidase Inhibitors	▪ Chronic gastro-intestinal disorders ▪ Cirrhosis, creatinine > 2.0	Periodic liver function tests (acarbose only)	No	Flatulence

Table 2.3 (continued on next page)

Dosage and cost			
	Typical starting cost (cost/month)	***Suggested maximum dose (cost/month)*** •	***Typical titration schedule***
Sulfonylureas			
Glipizide *	5mg QAM $ 9.58	10mg QAM $17.66	↑ 5mg Q week
Glipizide GITS (Glucotrol XL)	5mg QAM $10.65	10mg QAM $21.09	↑ 5mg Q week
Glyburide *	.5mg QAM $15.58	10mg QAM $31.17	↑ 2.5mg Q week
Glyburide,* micronized	3.0mg QAM $17.72	6mg QAM $25.23	↑ 3mg Q week
Glimepiride (Amaryl)	2mg QAM $11.98	4mg QAM $22.48	↑ 2mg Q weeks
Meglitinides			
Repaglinide	0.5mg TID AC $51.61	2mg TID AC $74.70	↑ 1-2mg/dose Q 1-2 weeks
Biguanides			
Metformin	500mg QD $19.39	1000mg BID AC $79.87	500mg QD x 2 wks 500mg BID x 2 wks 1GQAM & 50mg QPM x 2 wks 1G BID (all doses AC)
Thiazolidine-diones			
Rosiglitazone (Avandia)	4mg QD $75.00	4mg BID $150.00 or 8mg QD $136.90	↑ dose q 12 wks
Pioglitazone (Actos)	15mg QD $85.50	45mg QD $148.50	↑ dose q 12 wks

Dosing characteristics of sulfonylureas are shown in Table 2.3. Most (~75%) of the hypoglycemic action is observed with a daily dose that represents half of the maximally effective dose, that is, 10 mg of glyburide or glipizide or 4 mg of glimepiride.

The most common side effect of sulfonylureas is hypoglycemia (Table 2.2). The reported frequency of hypoglycemia with sulfonylureas, however, is low (2-5%), and side effects are usually mild and reversible upon discontinuation of therapy. As glycemic control improves to the near-normal range, the risk for hypoglycemia assumes greater importance. Hypoglycemia

Table 2.3 (cont'd)

Dosage and cost			
	Typical starting cost (cost/month)	***Recommended maximum dose (cost/month)*** ♦	***Typical titration schedule***
Alpha Glucose Inhibitors			
Acarbose (Precose)	25mg QD AC $15.51	50/100mg TID AC $46.54/$60.01	25mg QD x 2 wks 25mg BID x 2 wks 25mg TID x 2 wks Then double dose q2-4 wks.
Miglitol (Glyset)	25mg QD AC $14.63	50/100mg TID AC $51.75/$59.26	25mg QD x 2 wks 25mg BID x 2 wks 25mg TID x 2 wks Then double dose q2-4 wks.

★ Generic

♦ Slightly better results may be achieved if a higher dose is used

Average wholesale price courtesy of Redbook 2000

may be more severe and prolonged in high-risk groups, e.g., those who are elderly, likely to miss meals, have poor nutrition, or have concomitant hepatic, renal or cardiovascular disease. Moreover, the consequences of hypoglycemia may have greater consequences in certain groups, including patients with significant coronary heart disease. Hypoglycemic episodes in these patients with underlying coronary heart disease may precipitate ischemia. Many studies indicate that hypoglycemia is more common and severe with glyburide than the other sulfonylureas.

Notably, the sulfonylureas are the least expensive of all oral medications. In chronic disease states, improved compliance with medications may be associated with lower drug costs.

Meglitinides

Repaglinide is the only member of the meglitinide family currently approved for clinical use.

Repaglinide is a nonsulfonylurea insulin secretagogue (Fig. 2.3) that requires the presence of glucose for its action. Several possible binding sites for repaglinide have been found on beta cells, and one of them is the sulfonylurea receptor. It is not currently known whether the effects of repaglininde are additive to those of a sulfonylurea. Because of its pharmacokinetic behavior, its administration results in a brief and rapid release of insulin. Repaglinide therapy is therefore targeted for patients with primarily postprandial hyperglycemia and normal fasting glucose levels.

Efficacy and Metabolic Effects

When used as monotherapy, the decreases in FPG and HbA_{1c} are similar in repaglinide as with sulfonylureas.

Repaglinide has no significant effect on plasma lipid levels. Repaglinide therapy is associated with weight gain comparable to what has been found with sulfonylureas.

Clinical Use

Repaglinide is rapidly absorbed (0.5 to 1 hours) and displays rapid plasma elimination. Following from this, repaglinide is dosed three time daily, given 15 minutes before each meal (Table 2.3).

Adverse effects and safety issues are shown in Table 2.2. Hypoglycemia is the only adverse side effect that has been associated with use of repaglinide. Because of its shorter duration of action, it may be associated with less frequent and less severe hypoglycemia than seen with the sulfonylureas. Although some available data support this idea, additional data are needed to prove it unequivocally.

α-Phenylalanine Derivatives

Nateglinide is a new insulinotropic agent derived from α-phenylalanine. It is currently under investigation and will likely become available soon. Nateglinide is similar to repaglinide in that it stimulates early insulin secretion and is targeted toward reducing postprandial glucose levels.

Drugs That Improve Insulin Action

Biguanides

Metformin is the only biguanide that is available in the United States. Another drug in this class, phenformin, previously was approved for use in the U.S. but was removed from the market because of a significant incidence of lactic acidosis. Metformin differs structurally from phenformin and when used in patients with normal renal function is rarely associated with lactic acidosis. Metformin, which has been available since 1959, continues to be used worldwide because of its effectiveness and good safety record.

Metformin is thought to work primarily by improving insulin action in the liver and thereby decreasing hepatic glucose production. To a lesser degree, metformin also improves insulin action in the muscle and increases insulin-mediated glucose uptake (Fig. 2.3).

Efficacy and Metabolic Effects

Metformin and sulfonylureas are equally effective at improving glycemic control. Clinical trials have documented that metformin consistently lowers the FPG by 60-70 mg/dl and the HbA_{1c} by 1.5-2.0%. As with sulfonylureas, the decrease in FPG level from baseline with metformin is highly correlated with the starting plasma glucose level. For example, in patients with a FPG level of 300 mg/dl or more, the mean decrease is about 120 mg/dl.

Metformin has been reported to decrease plasma triglyceride levels and LDL cholesterol levels by about 10-15%. The magnitude of the decrease in triglycerides is related to the fasting triglyceride level. HDL cholesterol levels either increase slightly or do not change with metformin therapy. Weight gain does not occur, and most studies show modest weight loss – 2 to 3 kg – during the first six months of therapy.

Clinical Use

An example of a dosing schedule for metformin is presented in Table 2.3. Side effects can be minimized by administering the drug with meals and by initiating treatment with a low dose and increasing the dose slowly.

Adverse effects and safety issues are shown in Table 2.2. Because metformin does not stimulate insulin secretion, it does not cause hypoglycemia when used as monotherapy. The most common side effects of metformin include diarrhea, abdominal discomfort, anorexia, and occasionally a metallic taste in the mouth. The symptoms are dose related and occur in 20-30% of patients. These can be minimized by slow titration. Metformin can interfere with vitamin B_{12} absorption, but this is rarely of clinical significance. Extensive worldwide experience indicates that lactic acidosis is a rare complication (0.03 cases/1,000 patient years) and usually occurs when the drug is inappropriately prescribed. Metformin should not be used in patients with renal disease, congestive heart failure requiring pharmacological treatment, respiratory insufficiency, any hypoxemic condition, and severe infection. It should be used with caution in patients with liver disease or alcohol abuse. There is no need to discontinue the drug prior to radiographic contrast studies with contrast media, but the drug should be held after such studies (usually 24-48 hours) until it is clear that renal function has not been compromised by the study. Metformin should be discontinued during acute illnesses.

Thiazolidinediones

Thiazolidinediones are the newest class of oral agents to become available for clinical use. Troglitazone became available for clinical use in the U.S. in 1997. In March 2000 it was removed from the market because of concerns regarding liver toxicity. Two thiazolidinediones are currently available in the U.S. Rosiglitazone was released for clinical use in May of 1999, and pioglitazone was released in July of 1999. As of September 2000, there are no head-to-head clinical trials to compare the clinical effects of these two agents.

The primary action of thiazolidinediones is to enhance insulin sensitivity. Thiazolidinediones affect both liver and muscle (Fig. 2.3). Although their principle effect appears to be primarily on the muscle. It is likely that part of their stimulatory effect on muscle glucose uptake and inhibitory effect on hepatic glucose production is secondary to a decrease in plasma free fatty acid levels and associated free fatty acid oxidation. A frequent side effect is lower extremity edema.

Efficacy and Metabolic Effects

When used as monotherapy, average reductions in plasma glucose values with thiazolidinediones appear to be less than those seen with sulfonylureas, repaglinide and metformin (Table 2.1). Published reports indicate that HbA_{1c} values decrease approximately 1.0-1.2% in response to these agents. Patients who are naïve to antidiabetic drug treatment, and patients being treated with thiazolidinediones in combination with metformin, sulfonylureas or insulin, have greater reductions in HbA_{1c} values.

Similar to what was found with troglitazone, pioglitazone is associated with a reduction in plasma triglyceride levels. Rosiglitazone does not appear to affect plasma triglycerides. Both pioglitazone and rosiglitazone increase plasma LDL and HDL cholesterol levels. However, with treatment the LDL particle may become less susceptible to oxidation and hence, less atherogenic. All of the thiazolidinediones are associated with an increase in body weight, which is attributable to both edema and an increase in total body fat. It currently is unknown whether the effects on lipids, edema and body fat are class effects or whether there are differences between the agents on these parameters. The long-term cardiovascular effect of these drugs are unknown at this time.

Clinical Use

Dosing recommendations for rosiglitazone and pioglitazone are outlined in Table 2.3.

Adverse effects and safety issues are summarized in Table 2.2. Thiazolidinediones do not cause hypoglycemia when used as monotherapy. Thiazolidinediones are associated with fluid retention and the expansion of the plasma volume, which results clinically as edema and a decrease in the plasma hemoglobin level. The thiazolidinediones should be used with caution in patients with NYHA class III or IV cardiac status. Unlike troglitazone, which was removed from the market because of hepatic toxicity, pioglitazone and rosiglitazone do not seem to be associated with this problem. The reported incidence of elevated liver enzymes in patients treated with these agents are 0.25% and 0.2% respectively, which is similar to what was observed with placebo. However, given the experience with troglitazone, these agents should not be initiated in patients with transaminase levels > 2.5 times the upper limit of normal at baseline. It is recommended that the ALT be measured every other month in the first year of use with these agents and periodically thereafter. Thiazolidinediones should be used with caution in patients with elevations in transaminases.

Drugs That Modify Intestinal Absorption

α-Glucosidase Inhibitors

There are two available α-glucosidase inhibitors, acarbose and miglitol. Their clinical effects appear to be very similar.

The α-glucosidase inhibitors competitively inhibit the ability of enzymes in the small intestinal brush border to break down oligosaccarides and disaccharides into monosaccharides. Intestinal carbohydrate absorption is thereby delayed, resulting in a decrease in postprandial glucose levels (Fig. 2.3).

Efficacy and Metabolic Effects

The potency of α-glucosidase inhibitors is approximately half that of sulfonylureas, meglitinides and metformin (Table 2.1). As monotherapy, these agents decrease FPG level by 25-30 mg/dl and the HbA_{1c} level by 0.7% to 1.0%. They primarily affect the postprandial glucose, which is decreased by 40-50 mg/dl after meal ingestion. These drugs are most useful in patients with new-onset diabetes, which is characterized by mild fasting hyperglycemia but elevated postprandial hyperglycemia.

The α-glucosidase inhibitors are metabolically neutral. They have minimal effect on lipids, and do not significantly affect body weight.

Clinical Use

A typical dosing schedule is outlined in Table 2.3.

The major side effects of therapy are gastrointestinal (carbohydrate), i.e., abdominal fullness, borborygmi, flatulence and occasionally diarrhea (Table 2.2). These effects are dose and substrate (carbohydrate) related and tend to diminish with continued drug use. They can be minimized by titrating the dose upward very slowly. With very high levels of acarbose (200-300 mg three times a day), elevated serum transaminases have been reported. Abnormal liver function tests return to normal when the drug is discontinued. The α-glucosidase inhibitors are contraindicated in patients with inflammatory bowel disease. They are not recommended in patients with cirrhosis or serum creatinine >2.0. Hypoglycemia does not occur in patients taking these drugs as monotherapy. However, if hypoglycemia occurs when they are used with insulin or a sulfonylurea, the patient must be treated with glucose and not sucrose or complex carbohydrates. Glucose absorption is not affected by α-glucosidase treatment.

Combination Therapy with Oral Agents

Most patients will not achieve their target glycemic control on oral monotherapy either initially or after several years of treatment. If one oral antidiabetic agent does not lower glycemia to the target range, changing to a different agent rarely achieves better glycemic control. However, combining two oral agents with different mechanisms of action will result in improved glycemic control. Numerous combinations of two oral agents have been shown to have additive or potentiative effects in reducing the blood glucose. The use of three different oral antidiabetic agents, although appealing on an intellectual level, has few clinical data to validate it. Furthermore, the side effect profile and cost of combinations of three or more oral agents may limit their use.

Combined oral agent therapy will lose its effectiveness when endogenous insulin secretion becomes markedly deficient. At that point, the addition of insulin will be required.

Insulin Therapy

Excellent glycemic control can be achieved with intensive insulin therapy when given as monotherapy. Multiple studies, however, have failed to demonstrate consistent superiority of insulin monotherapy over oral agents in controlling the blood sugar. Furthermore, weight gain directly related to the dose of insulin and hypoglycemia are common side effects of insulin. For these reasons insulin therapy for type 2 diabetes is usually reserved for treatment of patients in whom acceptable glycemic control does not occur with oral agents alone or in combination.

Multiple studies also have failed to demonstrate benefits of multiple injections of insulin compared with insulin given once a day. Addition of a bedtime (~9 pm) intermediate acting insulin, such as NPH (or the new insulin analogue, glargine, which is scheduled for release in the U.S. soon), to oral medication regimens is a safe and effective way of normalizing the day-long glycemic profile while minimizing weight gain and reducing insulin dose by 50-60% compared with a multiple dose insulin regimen.

Although oral agents used alone or in combination with insulin is the preferred initial therapy for patients with type 2 diabetes, it is common to encounter patients with poorly controlled type 2 diabetes on high dose insulin monotherapy. Addition of an oral agent that improves insulin action may be beneficial in these patients. The primary goal would be to improve the day-long glycemic profile (HbA_{1c} <7.0%). Addition of an oral agent also may allow the reduction in the dose of insulin, the number of injections or both.

Treatment Strategy

Figure 2.4 provides a general treatment strategy for patients with type 2 diabetes. In most patients whose disease is inadequately controlled with diet and exercise, pharmacologic therapy with a single oral agent should be initiated. The choice of agent should be a dictated by considerations of efficacy in lowering blood glucose, metabolic effects, and dose, safety and cost issues. Insulin may be indicated as initial therapy if patients are markedly symptomatic, if the fasting plasma glucose level is very high (>280-300 mg/dl), or if there is ketonuria or ketonemia. The dose of oral agent should be quickly increased until adequate glycemic control is achieved. The patient may be seen at 2-4 week intervals or more frequently as the dose is being titrated.

In patients whose disease is inadequately controlled with a single oral agent, a second oral agent, with a different mechanism of action, should be added. If glycemic control is inadequate with combination therapy with two oral agents, there are several possibilities. Bedtime intermediate-acting insulin (e.g. 10-15 units

Figure 2.4

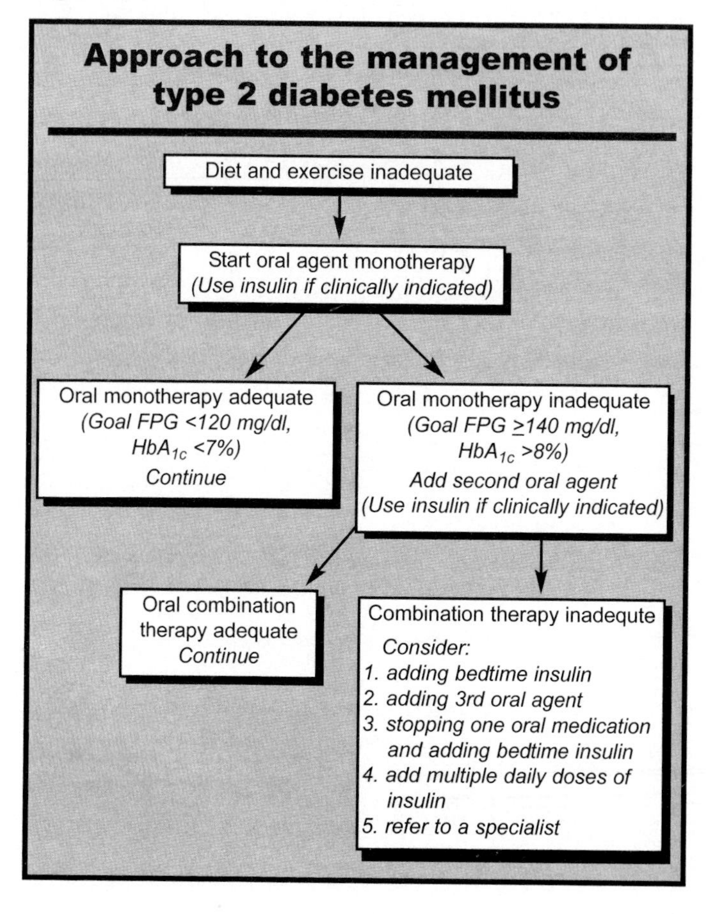
Approach to the management of type 2 diabetes mellitus
Diet and exercise inadequate
Start oral agent monotherapy
(Use insulin if clinically indicated)
Oral monotherapy adequate
(Goal FPG <120 mg/dl,
HbA1c <7%)
Continue
Oral monotherapy inadequate
(Goal FPG ≥140 mg/dl,
HbA1c >8%)
Add second oral agent
(Use insulin if clinically indicated)
Oral combination
therapy adequate
Continue
Combination therapy inadequte
Consider:
1. adding bedtime insulin
2. adding 3rd oral agent
3. stopping one oral medication and adding bedtime insulin
4. add multiple daily doses of insulin
5. refer to a specialist

NPH) may be added, a third oral agent may be added, or the patient may be changed to a more complex insulin regimen. At this point it would be reasonable to refer to a diabetes specialist.

In patients on insulin monotherapy (Fig. 2.5), addition of an oral agent to the regimen may improve glycemic control or allow a reduction in the insulin dose or number of injections. Metformin, a thiazolidinedione or α-glucosidase inhibitor may be added to the current insulin regimen. Another commonly used regimen consists of the combination of a sulfonylurea given in the morning with insulin given before dinner or before bedtime. When daytime insulin is required, the addition of an insulin secretagogue probably will not be useful.

Figure 2.5

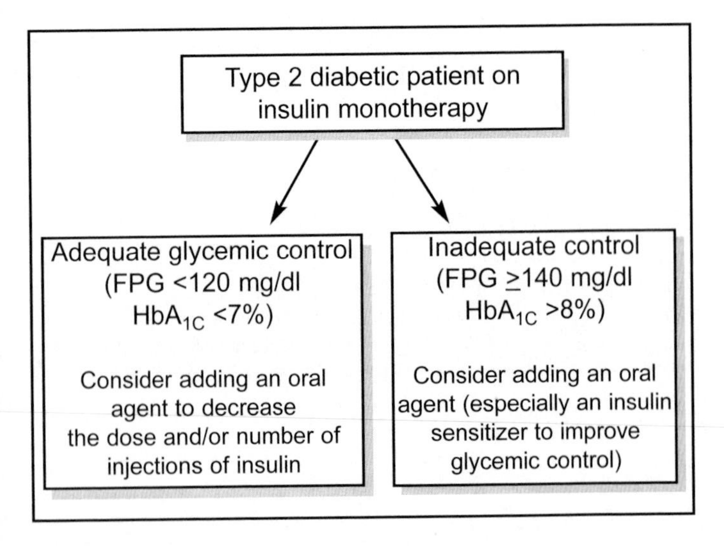

Table 2.4

Cost of insulin therapy per bottle	
(1,000 units per bottle: one bottle lasts one month in a patient taking 33 units per day of selected product)	
Humulin NPH	$20.60
Novolin NPH	$20.60
Humulin reg	$20.60
Novolin reg	$20.60
Humalog	$28.50
B-D insulin syringes (box of 100)	$26.00
Home blood glucose test strips	$1-2 per strip
Prices listed as Average Wholesale Price courtesy of Xavier University D.I.C.	

Selected References:

1. DeFronzo, Ralph A. Pharmacological therapy for type 2 diabetes mellitus. Ann Intern Med. 1999;131:281-303.
2. Therapy for Diabetes and Related Disorders, third edition. Editor, Harold E. Lebovitz. The American Diabetes Association, Inc., 1998.
3. UK Prospective Diabetes Study (UKPDS) Group. Intensive blood-glucose control with sulphomylureas or insulin compared with conventional treatment and risk of complications in patients with type 2 diabetes (UKPDS 33). Lancet 1998; 352-837.
4. Turner RC, Cull CA, Frighi V, Holman RR for the UK Prospective Diabetes Study (UKPDS) Group. Glycemic control with diet, sulfonylurea, metformin, or insulin inpatients with type 2 diabetes. Progressive requirement for multiple therapies (UKPDS 49). JAMA 1999; 281: 2005.

5. DeFronzo RA, Goodman AM, and the Multicenter Metformin Study Group. Efficacy of metformin in patients with non-insulin-dependent diabetes mellitus. N Engl J Med 1995; 333:541.
6. Wolffenbuttel BHR, Landgraf R, et al. A one-year multicenter randomized double-blind comparison of repaglinide and glyburide for the treatment of type 2 diabetes. Diabetes Care 1999; 22:463.
7. Moses R, Slobodniuk R, Boyages S. et al. Effect of repaglinide addition to metformin monotherapy on glycemic control in patients with type 2 diabetes. Diabetes Care 1999; 22:119.
8. Chaisson JL, Josse RG, Hunt JA, et al.The efficacy of acarbose inthe treatment of patients with non-insulin-dependent diabetes mellitus. A multicenter controlled clinical trial. Ann Intern Med 1994; 121:928.
9. Yki-Jarvinen H, Kauppila M, Kujansuu E, et al. Comparison of insulin regimens inpatients with non-insulin-dependent diabtetes mellitus. N Engl J Med 1992; 327:1426.
10. Yki-JSrvinen H, Ryssy L, NikkilS K, et al. Comparison of bedtime insulin regimens in patients with type 2 diabetes mellitus. A randomized controlled trial. Ann Intern Med 1999; 130:389.

Diagnostic Evaluation for Coronary Artery Disease in the Patient with Diabetes Mellitus

Gary E. Sander, MD, PhD

Atherosclerosis in Diabetes

The manifestations of diabetic heart disease include atherosclerosis, cardiomyopathy and diabetic autonomic neuropathy; the pathophysiologic process includes macrovascular disease, microvascular disease, myocellular hypertrophy and fibrosis, and autonomic nerve fiber degeneration. These multiple processes make the precise definition of coronary artery status difficult in the individual with diabetes, regardless of the presence or absence of symptoms. However, cardiovascular disease, including coronary artery disease (CAD), cerebrovascular disease, and peripheral vascular disease, is the most common cause of death in diabetic patients; the majority of deaths result from CAD (1,2,3). Despite the premature occurrence of CAD in diabetic patients, the more extensive disease at diagnosis, the greater morbidity and mortality after infarction, and the reduced success with revascularization, histopathological studies have indicated similarity in plaque composition and structure between diabetic and non-diabetic individuals (4,5,6). However, diabetic atherosclerotic plaques are often more diffuse and distal in distribution; small vessel disease and endothelial dysfunction with resultant blunted vasodilatory responses are present as well. Further, CAD is frequently silent in diabetes. Silent myocardial ischemia is found in 10 to 20% of the diabetic population as compared to 1 to 4% of non-diabetics (6,7,8).

Rationale for Testing

The possibility in the diabetic patient of a large but asymptomatic ischemic burden, coupled with the poor outcome in diabetic patients following myocardial infarction, make it imperative to seek effective means of early identification of coronary disease in the diabetic patient. General indications for cardiac testing are listed in Table 3.1 and will be considered in more detail in subsequent sections. In light of recent suggestions that all diabetic patients be treated to secondary prevention targets and that aspirin and ACE inhibitors be administered early, it is possible that medical management may not change significantly. Thus the challenge is to identify

Table 3.1

Indications for testing for asymptomatic CAD
1. ECG consistent with ischemia
2. Peripheral or carotid obstructive vascular disease
3. Age >65 years with duration of type 2 diabetes >10 years
4. Plans to begin a vigorous exercise program
5. Evaluation before renal transplantation
6. Preoperative clearance for major vascular or non-cardiac surgery
7. Atypical cardiac symptoms
8. Two or more of the following risk factors in addition to diabetes:
■ total cholesterol ≥240 mg/dl; LDL-c ≥160 mg/dl; or HDL-c <35 mg/dl
■ blood pressure >140/90 mmHg
■ cigarette smoking
■ positive family history of premature CAD
■ positive micro/macroalbuminuria test

asymptomatic patients needing revascularization, and by early identification and treatment, reduce the rate of subsequent cardiovascular events. Medical interventions with control of blood pressure and dyslipidemia, together with appropriate revascularization, have led to significant reductions in cardiovascular morbidity and mortality in this group.

In order to provide some guidance for physicians concerning cardiac testing of both symptomatic and asymptomatic diabetic patients, the American Diabetes Association and the American College of Cardiology (ADA-ACC) held a Consensus Development Conference in February 1998. The consensus position has been published (6) and is further elaborated in this chapter.

Selection of Diagnostic Tests

The selection of initial screening tests should be governed by the intent of testing: to detect occult disease or to estimate prognosis and provide risk-stratification. Those pathophysiological processes present in diabetes cause biochemical and physiological changes which alter the sensitivity, specificity and interpretation of non-invasive testing. The major factors are listed in Table 3.2 and discussed in more detail elsewhere (9). Additionally, these factors may result in poor exercise performance levels, which will also reduce the sensitivity of testing. More expensive testing, such as SPECT sestamibi imaging, may be required. The ECG itself is a very inexpensive and useful tool. A normal ECG virtually precludes the presence of significant systolic dysfunction (10). On the other hand, ST-T abnormalities on the resting ECG have been identified as a significant risk factor in both men and women for the subsequent demonstration of asymptomatic CAD by exercise ECG and thallium-201 (^{201}Tl) scintigraphy (11). In the diabetic patient who is able to exercise and has a normal or near normal ECG, a simple treadmill or bicycle exercise test, evaluating exercise capacity, ventricular reserve, and ST segment changes, will detect almost all patients with left main and significant three vessel disease. A normal test indicates a good prognosis. In a prospective study of 110 insulin-requiring diabetic subjects with no clinical evidence of cardiac disease, the peak treadmill heart rate was the single most important predictor of the subsequent development of clinical coronary heart disease; all of the 14 patients who experienced a cardiac event had a

Table 3.2

Factors producing false positive screening tests in diabetic patients	
Comorbidity	***Pathophysiologic consequence***
Hypertension	↑ LVM → false positive ETT, ^{201}T1 defects
Cardiomyopathy	Wall motion abnormalities, blunted adrenergic enhancement of contractility, ^{201}T1 defects
Renal disease	↑ adenosine concentration → ↓ maximal flow reserve following dipyridamole → ↓ sensitivity of scintigraphy
Autonomic neuropathy	↓ chronotropic response to exercise, ↓ coronary vasodilator capacity, dissociation of cardiac from external work
Endothelial dysfunction	↓ coronary vasodilator capacity

treadmill result that was either abnormal or inconclusive due to failure to achieve 90% of the predicted maximal heart rate. Conversely, no patient with a normal treadmill test result experienced a cardiac event in the subsequent 50-month period (12).

In another study of 59 middle-aged diabetic patients with suspected coronary artery disease, sensitivity and specificity for maximal ECG exercise test was 75% and 77%, respectively, for significant CAD (≥70% occlusion of at least one coronary artery); this compared with sensitivity and specificity of 80% and 87% for ^{201}Tl myocardial scintigraphy, and only 25% and 88% for ambulatory ECG monitoring (13). Perfusion imaging with ^{201}Tl or technicium-99m (^{99m}Tc) sestamibi, preferably with exercise but also effective with pharmacological vasodilation, allows quantification of the extent of perfusion abnormalities which are important in both identifying the presence of disease and providing prognostic information. Multiple perfusion defects, large defects or areas of reversibility, reduced ventricular function, increased isotope uptake in the lung, and transient left ventricular dilation are all predictive of future cardiac events. In patients with angiographically "normal" coronary arteries, abnormal perfusion scans may indicate diffuse coronary disease or endothelial dysfunction and an increased event rate relative to individuals with normal perfusion scans.

Stress echocardiography is a reasonable alternative to stress perfusion imaging in the presence of appropriate echocardiographic expertise. Perfusion imaging is superior to stress echocardiography in the detection of single vessel disease and in detecting ischemia; techniques are similar in ability to detect multivessel disease. The role of dobutamine stress echocardiographic (DSE) testing appears very limited at this time. A dissociation between myocardial oxidative metabolism (demonstrated by ^{11}C-acetate clearance by PET scanning) and cardiac work (rate-pressure-product) has been demonstrated in type 2 diabetic patients with normal stress-perfusion SPECT; this defect in myocardial oxidative metabolism becomes apparent during dobutamine stress (14). Furthermore, infusion of dobutamine into young insulin-dependent diabetic subjects (mean age 28.5 years) with normal myocardial contractile reserves uncovers defective and blunted recruitment of myocardial contractility which is strongly related to impairment of cardiac sympathetic innervation as confirmed by ^{123}I-metaiodobenzylguanidine (MIBG) scintigraphy (15). The sensitivity, specificity, positive and negative predictive values of DSE for detection of asymptomatic CAD in 52 type 2 diabetic patients (mean age 59 years) are 82%, 54%, 84%, and 50%, respectively (16). Similar results have been reported in asymptomatic type one diabetic patients with nephropathy (17). Thirty-eight percent of 18 patients had results suggestive of ischemia; 17% also had significant dysrhythmias. Coronary angiography performed in six of the seven subjects with positive DSE demonstrated significant CAD in only two. In yet another study in which the prognostic value of DSE performed early after acute myocardial infarction was assessed in both diabetic and non-diabetic patients, positive DSE results were associated with a lower event-free survival rate in non-diabetic but not in diabetic patients; in diabetic patients a shorter dobutamine time, rather than a positive DSE result, independently predicted cardiac events (18). On the other hand, DSE was helpful in predicting cardiac events in a group of 53 type 1 diabetic patients undergoing evaluation for kidney and/or pancreas transplantation; event rates were 45% among those with an abnormal, versus 6% among those with a normal, DSE (19). Thus the role of DSE in assessing asymptomatic diabetic patients appears very limited.

Testing in Symptomatic Heart Disease

"Symptomatic" cardiac disease in the diabetic individual may include typical angina; it has been reported that over 15% of type 2 diabetic patients over age 65 have angina. Atypical symptoms include dyspnea, fatigue, and gastrointestinal complaints with exertion. Individuals with such complaints require further evaluation to determine etiology of symptoms and type of cardiac disease which may be present, the need for invasive testing, and the most appropriate therapeutic intervention. Unexplained congestive heart failure, particularly when resulting from systolic left ventricular dysfunction, requires testing to exclude asymptomatic CAD. However, the majority of diabetic patients presenting with coronary artery disease as the cause of systolic heart failure will have ECG evidence of ischemia, often Q waves indicative of prior myocardial infarction. Assessment of myocardial perfusion and regional ventricular function with exercise ^{99m}Tc sestamibi gated SPECT imaging has been reported to reliably distinguish between patients with ischemic cardiomyopathy and patients with non-ischemic cardiomyopathy. SPECT imaging may have application in the diabetic population as well (20). As suggested in Figure 3.1, derived from the ADA-ACC consensus conference, the test selection is determined by the severity of symptoms and the presence and extent of ECG abnormalities which could either limit the ability to interpret a routine exercise stress test or indicate more extensive heart disease, such as prior myocardial infarction, than suggested clinically. Those patients with symptoms suggestive of moderate or more severe angina or ECG evidence of CAD, particularly if associated with heart failure, will in most cases benefit from cardiac catheterization without prior screening in order to quickly establish the presence and extent of atherosclerosis and to allow prompt initiation of appropriate treatment.

Testing in Asymptomatic Heart Disease

There have been several attempts to define the prevalence of asymptomatic CAD, defined by a myocardial scar or demonstrable reversible ischemia without chest pain or anginal equivalent (Table 3.3). The Milan Study on Atherosclerosis and Diabetes (MiSAD) group found ischemic ST segment responses by exercise testing in 12% of 925 type 2 diabetic

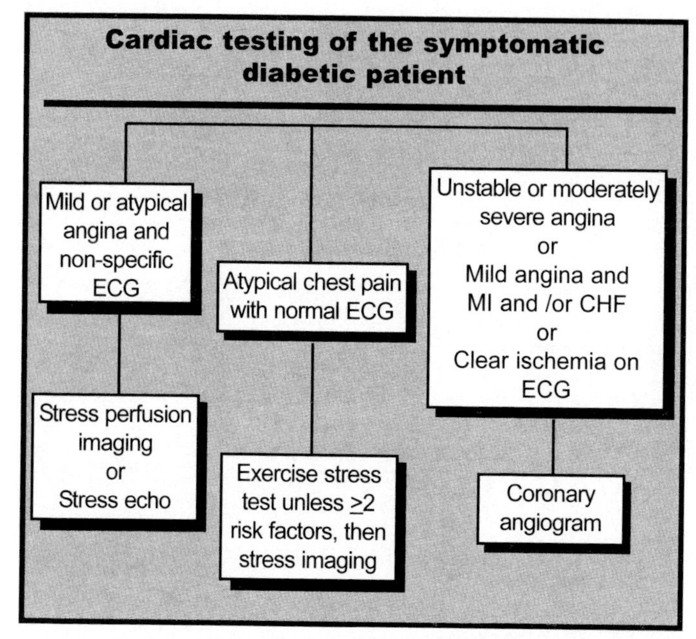

Figure 3.1. Cardiac testing of the symptomatic diabetic patient. This algorithm provides a testing sequence for diabetic patients presenting with atypical chest pain or overt evidence of cardiovascular disease which is likely ischemic in etiology. Those patients who cannot exercise should be tested by pharmacological stress testing with thallium −201 or technicium −99m sestamibi (6).

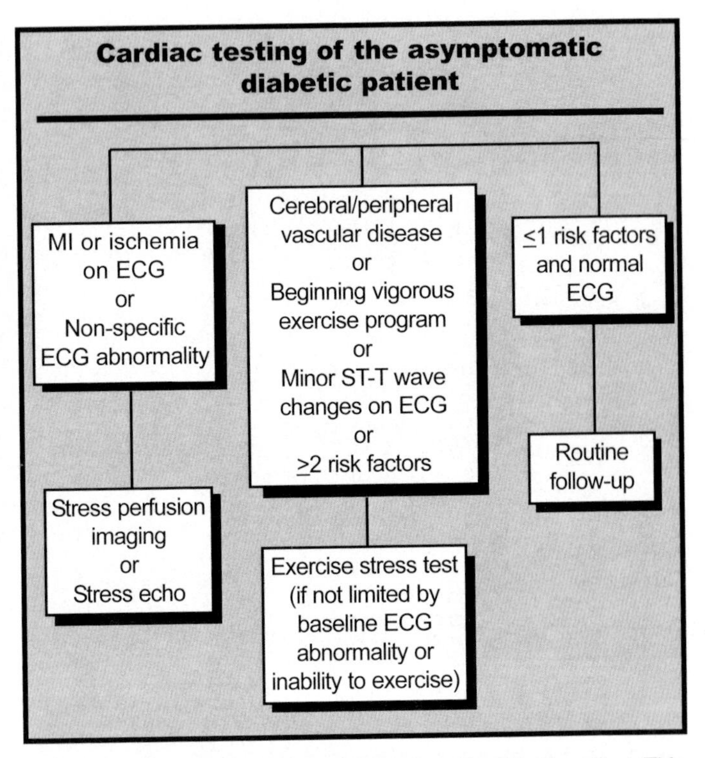

Figure 3.2. Cardiac testing of the asymptomatic diabetic patient. This algorithm provides a testing sequence for asymptomatic diabetic patients based upon the presence and severity of risk factors and co-existing atherosclerotic vascular disease or ECG abnormalities. As in the case of symptomatic patients, those patients who cannot exercise should be tested by pharmacological stress testing with thallium −201 or technicium −99m sestamibi (6).

patients treated with either oral hypoglycemic agents or diet; 59 of these 112 (53%) also had positive ^{201}Tl scintigraphy, representing 6% of the total population. No angiographic confirmation was performed (11). In another study with angiographic confirmation, positive exercise test results were observed in 31% of 132 type 2 diabetic patients (21); 36 out of the 41 patients with positive tests had significant CAD, representing 11% of the total population. A third study described similar results: a 29% positive screening rate and a 6% rate of significant CAD confirmed by angiography (8). In this study, described earlier, all screened patients underwent angiography; only 30% of those with a positive noninvasive screening test had documented CAD, again supporting the observation that a positive noninvasive screening test has a low positive predictive value.

Indications for testing truly asymptomatic diabetic patients are listed in Table 3.1. The benefits should be most apparent in groups exposed to periods of high cardiac risk, such as those planned for renal transplantation, high risk non-cardiac or vascular surgery, and

Table 3.3

Incidence of asymptomatic CAD in diabetic patients		
Study (ref)	*+ Screening test (% total)*	*+ CAD (% total)*
MiSAD (12)	+ ETT in 112/925 (12%)	+ ^{201}T1 scintigraphy in 59/112 (6%)
Koistinen (8)	+ Holter, ETT and/or ^{201}T1 scintigraphy in 40/136 (29%)	+ CAD by angiogram in 12/34 (6%)
Naka (22)	+ ETT in 41/132 (31%)	+ CAD by angiogram in 14/36 (11%)

those initiating a vigorous exercise program. The ADA-ACC testing algorithm is depicted in Figure 3.2. As described earlier, the predictive value of the ECG alone is adequate such that diabetic patients with one or fewer risk factors and a normal ECG do not require cardiac testing, but simple routine surveillance. Exercise stress testing alone is appropriate unless the ability to interpret this test is limited by baseline ECG abnormality or inability of the patient to exercise to 85% of the maximum predicted heart rate. The inability to achieve the target heart rate, which may be influenced by the presence of autonomic neuropathy, renders a negative test indeterminate. In the presence of an indeterminate outcome, testing should be repeated using pharmacological stress imaging.

A group of French investigators have reported the results obtained by following a very similar set of guidelines promulgated by the Association de Langue Francaise pour l'Etude du Diabete et des Maladies Metaboliques, or ALFEDIAM (22). Inclusion criteria were age between 25 and 75, duration of diabetes (>15 years type 1, >10 years type 2 with no risk factors, >5 years type 2 with ≥1 risk factor), and absence of clinical or ECG evidence of CAD. Over the first year of study, 203 patients were screened using the protocol outlined in Figure 3.3. Exercise ECG was the first choice for screening method. If exercise ECG was not possible or inconclusive (<95% of the maximal predicted rate for age), ^{201}Tl myocardial scintigraphy with exercise testing and/or dipyridamole was performed. If either of these tests was positive, then angiography was performed and was considered positive in the presence of ≥50% stenosis. Positive screening results occurred in 32% of patients (15.7%). Twenty-six patients subsequently underwent angiography; significant lesions were demonstrated in 19 patients (9.3% of total population, 76% of test group) and non-significant lesions in seven patients (one false positive result for exercise ECG and six false

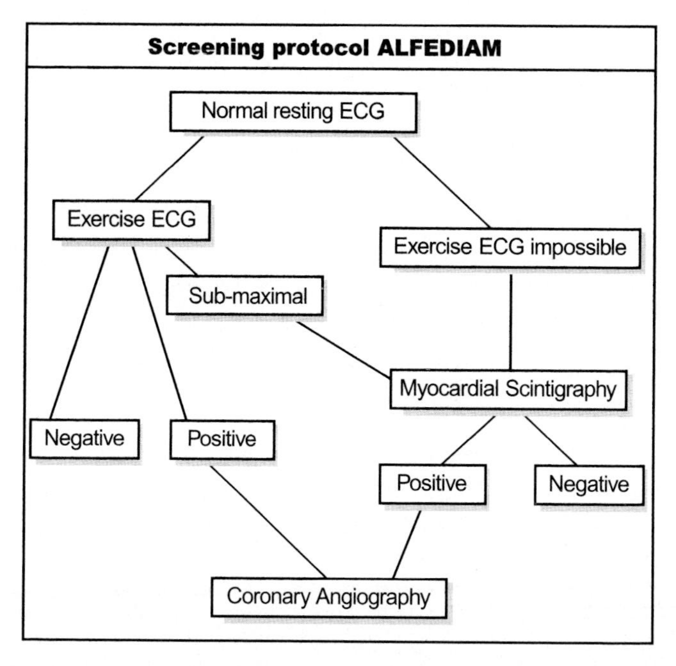

Figure 3.3. The screening protocol used by the Association de Langue Francaise pour l'Etude du Diabete et des Maladies Metaboliques (ALFEDIAM). Exercise ECG was considered submaximal if the patient failed to achieve 95% of the maximal predicted heart rate for age. Myocardial scintigraphy was performed by dipyridamole-^{201}Tl technique (23).

positive results for ^{201}Tl scintigraphy). In this small experimental group, the positive predictive value was 90% for the exercise ECG and 62.5% for ^{201}Tl scintigraphy. Of the 19 patients (15 men, 4 women) with asymptomatic CAD, 16 presented with type 2 diabetes. The main differences between the 16 type 2 diabetic patients with asymptomatic CAD and the type 2 diabetic patients without asymptomatic CAD were a higher prevalence of peripheral macroangiopathy (56.2% versus 15.1%) and a high prevalence of retinopathy. Asymptomatic CAD occurred in 20.9% of type 2 male diabetic patients who met the entry criteria for this study. No correlations were found between asymptomatic CAD and duration of diabetes, extent of glucose control, renal status, or cardiovascular risk factors except for family history of CAD. The authors concluded that since 20.9% of asymptomatic male patients with type 2 diabetes have evidence of asymptomatic CAD and since there is a high positive predictive value of functional testing, routine screening for asymptomatic CAD would be useful in this patient subgroup.

Coronary artery disease is particularly common in individuals with established peripheral vascular disease. Seventeen of 30 diabetic patients (57%) without clinical suspicion of coronary artery disease were found to have abnormal dipyridamole ^{201}Tl scintigraphy; reversible defects compatible with ischemia appeared in 14 patients (47%) and evidence of prior clinically silent myocardial infarction in 11 patients (47%). These abnormalities were most frequent in patients with hypertension and cigarette smoking (23). Since cardiovascular complications represent a major risk to patients undergoing vascular surgery, these investigators then evaluated 101 diabetic patients with dipyridamole-^{201}Tl scintigraphy prior to surgery. Eighty percent of the overall group displayed ^{201}Tl abnormalities which did not correlate with clinical markers of coronary disease; 59% of the subgroup of patients with no overt clinical evidence of underlying heart disease had abnormal scans. Cardiovascular complications occurred in 11% of all patients. The quantification of the total number of reversible defects and assessment of ischemia in the distribution of the left anterior descending coronary artery were required for optimal predictive accuracy (24).

Significance of Positive Screening Results

Those studies described in the previous section were designed to detect the presence and prevalence of asymptomatic CAD. As stated earlier, the ultimate justification for such screening depends upon whether or not detection of CAD will alter management in such a way as to reduce cardiovascular morbidity and mortality (9). There has been an attempt to determine the prognostic value of the exercise stress test and ^{201}Tl SPECT scintigraphy for the prediction of cardiac events in a selected high risk group of type 2 diabetic patients (Fig. 3.4) (25). This group included 158 patients (105 men aged 63±9 years) with two or more of the following characteristics: age ≥65 years, active smoking, hypertension >160/95 mm Hg, hypercholesterolemia (cholesterol >219 mg/dl or LDL >120 mg/dl), peripheral vascular disease, abnormal resting ECG, or microalbuminuria (20-200 μg/min). Exercise stress scintigraphy was performed in 77 patients able to exercise on an ergometer bicycle to achieve ≥85% of the maximum predicted heart rate for age; dipyridamole scintigraphy was performed in 80 patients unable to exercise. Causes of the inability to exercise

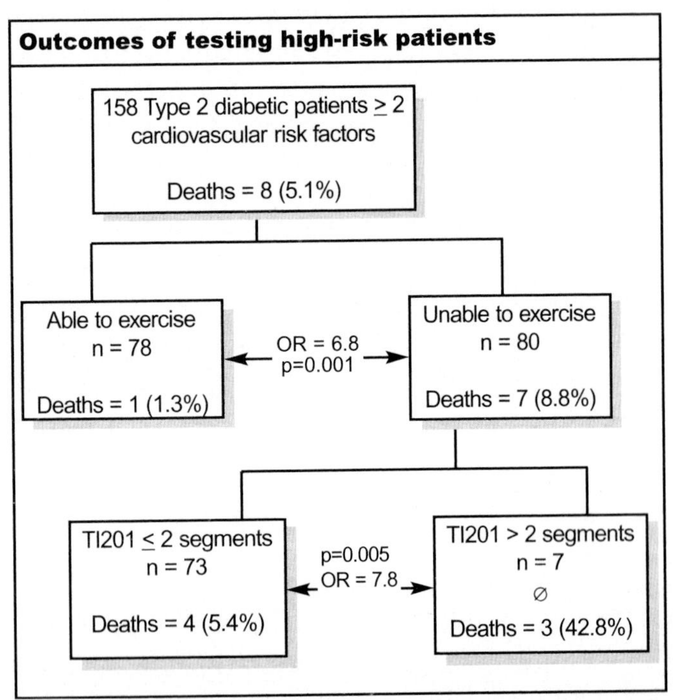

Figure 3.4. The incremental prognostic value over 23 ± 7 months of follow-up afforded by the use of ^{201}Tl SPECT scanning in high-risk diabetic patients unable to exercise on a bicycle ergometer to 85% of the maximum predicted heart rate for age (25).

included obesity, chronic fatigue, peripheral neuropathy, pulmonary disease, peripheral vascular disease, congestive heart failure, or previous cerebrovascular accident. Subjects were followed for 23 ± 7 months; the annual event rate was 7.3%, including eight deaths and 14 myocardial infarctions. Independent predictors of events included age >60 years, abnormal resting ECG, microalbuminuria, the inability to exercise, and the presence of more than two defects detected by scintigraphy. Cardiac death occurred in 1.3% of patients able to exercise versus 8.8% of patients unable to exercise; in this latter group large perfusion defects corresponded with an annual mortality rate of 22.3%. The number of reversible defects predicted future myocardial infarction, while fixed defects, indicating irreversibly injured myocardium and altered left ventricular function, were related to the occurrence of future cardiac death. A coronary angiogram was performed on 25 patients (6 after myocardial infarction, eight after development of unstable angina, eight for typical or atypical chest pain, and three before major non-cardiac surgery); 8, 6, 6, and 5 patients had no, one-, two-, and three-vessel disease (stenosis >50%). Only eight patients were judged to need myocardial revascularization. In this very high risk population, the negative predictive value of a normal ^{201}Tl scintigraphy study for major cardiac events and death was 94% and 97%, respectively.

In a study very similar to those described in the previous section, the predictive role of dipyridamole ^{201}Tl scanning in identifying perioperative cardiovascular events has been further tested in patients both with (Group B) and without (Group A) clinical evidence of cardiac disease (26). Scans were abnormal in 58% of 36 Group A patients and 93% of 57 Group B patients. When compared with Group B patients with perfusion defects, Group A patients with perfusion abnormalities had fewer defects per scan (2.7 ± 1.5 vs 3.6 ± 1.9); despite the presence of defects, no perioperative cardiac complications occurred in Group A patients but nine of 57 Group B patients experienced events. However, in this study preoperative imaging added little to the clinical assessment for evidence of cardiac disease.

Furthermore, in the ALFEDIAM study described earlier, despite identification of asymptomatic CAD in 19 patients, only seven underwent revascularization, all with percutaneous techniques. Similarly, in the group of 158 high-risk diabetic patients described earlier, only eight required revascularization.

Appropriate Follow-up of Screening Tests

As suggested in Table 3.4, diabetic patients with normal stress tests need no further evaluation, but continue to require close surveillance for changes in clinical state. Routine follow-up should include annual ECG and screening for signs and symptoms of CAD or left ventricular dysfunction. The exercise treadmill test should generally be repeated in three to five years or earlier if there is deterioration in clinical status. Closer follow-up, such as a repeat of the exercise treadmill test in one to two years, is indicated in high-risk situations. Individuals with "markedly" positive stress tests, defined by such features as hypotension during exercise, a positive test at heart rate <110 bpm, exercise capacity <6 minutes (<Stage 2 of standard Bruce protocol or < 5 METS), ST segment depression in ≥5 leads, or >2 mm maximum ST segment depression, should undergo coronary angiography if at all possible. Asymptomatic patients with "mildly" positive stress tests, such as 1-1.5 mm ST segment depression at a moderate to high exercise level (≥Bruce Stage 3) are generally at relatively low risk; perfusion imaging or stress echocardiography should be utilized to exclude false positive ECG responses. Perfusion imaging should be considered in moderate to high-risk individuals because further risk stratification may be warranted. Even in those individuals with moderately positive ECG stress tests, normal to near

Table 3.4

Appropriate follow-up after screening test

Pre-test risk	***ETT results***			
	Normal	***Mildly positive***	***Moderately positive***	***Markedly positive***
High (≥RF)	2	3	4	4
Moderate (2-3 RF)	1	3	3	4
Low (≤1 RF)	1	3	3	4

1. Routine follow-up: yearly ECG, repeat ETT in 3-5 years
2. Close follow-up: repeat ETT in 1-2 years
3. Nuclear or echocardiographic imaging study
4. Coronary angiogram

(Risk factors are those listed in Table 3.1)

normal perfusion studies indicate a very good prognosis (<2 percent annual cardiac event rate); conversely moderate to large perfusion defects indicate significant risk of cardiac events over the next one to two years and identify patients who should undergo coronary angiography and possible revascularization.

Conclusions

It is apparent that in the asymptomatic diabetic patient, the clinical status itself is very important in predicting the presence of asymptomatic CAD. The asymptomatic patient with a normal ECG, and particularly with a normal exercise ECG, is at very low risk for cardiovascular events and simply requires periodic medical evaluation. The patient with abnormal screening tests requires more comprehensive evaluation, which should be planned in light of the poor positive predictive value of currently available screening tests in this population. It is estimated that up to 6% of the population may suffer from type 2 diabetes mellitus. Thus the diagnostic evaluation should be designed to provide optimal value; it is imperative to utilize resources in such a way as to maximize the benefits for costs expended. The target group for which an aggressive detection strategy is most cost effective are males with type 2 diabetics, aged 65 or greater, and with associated risk factors. Those diabetic patients with associated disease processes, including complications of diabetes, also require very careful assessment. Other individuals should be selected on an individual basis, utilizing such factors as overall clinical status, exercise performance, and extent of damaged or compromised myocardium as demonstrated by isotope scanning. Those individuals then demonstrated by angiography to have significant CAD can then be directed to appropriate revascularization with anticipated prolongation of survival. Furthermore, those diabetic patients identified as having asymptomatic CAD will benefit from more aggressive medical management; treatment goals will shift from primary prevention interventions to those of secondary prevention. Conversely, since the negative predictive value is high, testing may be helpful in excluding silent ischemia in situations of anticipated high physiological stress, such as major noncardiac surgery.

References:

1. Kannel WB, McGee DL. Diabetes and cardiovascular disease: the Framingham Study. JAMA 1979;241:2035-8.
2. UK Prospective Diabetes Study Group: Intensive blood-glucose control with conventional treatment and risk of complications in patients with type 2 diabetes (UKPDS 33). Lancet 1998;352:837-853.
3. Fuller JH. Mortality trends and causes of death in diabetic patients. Diabet Metab 1993;38:726-31.
4. Jacoby RM, Nesto RW. Acute myocardial infarction in the diabetic patient: pathophysiology, clinical course and prognosis. J Am Coll Cardiol 1992;20:736-44.
5. Fava S, Azzopardi J, Muscat HA, Fenech FF. Factors that influence outcome in diabetic subjects with myocardial infarction. Diabetes Care 1993;16:1615-18.
6. American Diabetes Association. Consensus development

conference on the diagnosis of coronary heart disease in people with diabetes. Diabetes Care 1998;21:1551-59.

7. Nesto RW, Phillips RT, Kett KG, Hill T, Perper E, Young E, Leland OS. Relationship of angina to ischemia in diabetics and nondiabetics: assessment by exercise thallium scintigraphy. Ann Intern Med 1988;108:170-75.
8. Koistinen MJ. Prevalence of asymptomatic myocardial ischemia in diabetic subjects. BMJ 1990;301:92-5.
9. Nesto RW. Screening for asymptomatic coronary artery disease in diabetes. Diabetes Care 1999;22:1393-5.
10. Talreju D, Gruver C, Sklenar J, Dent J, Kaul S. Efficient utilization of echocardiography for the assessment of left ventricular systolic function. Am Heart J 2000;139:394-8.
11. Milan Study on Atherosclerosis and Diabetes (MiSAD) Group: Prevalence of unrecognized silent myocardial ischemia and its association with atherosclerotic risk factors in non insulin-dependent diabetes mellitus. Am J Cardiol 1997; 79:134-9.
12. Gerson MC, Khoury JC, Hertzberg VS, Fischer EE, Scott RC. Prediction of coronary artery disease in a population of insulin-requiring diabetic patients: results of an 8-year follow-up study. Am Heart J 1988;116:820-6.
13. Paillole C, Ruiz J, Juliard JM, Leblanc H, Gourgon R, Passa P. Detection of coronary artery disease in diabetic patients. Diabetologia 1995;38:726-31.
14. Hattori N, Tamaki N, Kudoh T, Magata Y, Kitano H, Inubushi M, Tadamura E, Nakao K, Konishi J. Abnormality of myocardial oxidative metabolism in non insulin-dependent diabetes mellitus. J Nucl Med 1998;39:1835-40.
15. Scognamiglio R, Avogaro A, Casara D, Crepaldi C, Marin M, Palisi M, Mingardi R, Erle G, Fasoli G, Dalla Volta S. Myocardial dysfunction and adrenergic cardiac innervation in patients with insulin-dependent diabetes mellitus. J Am Coll Cardiol 1998;31:404-12.
16. Hennessy TG, Codd MB, Kane G, McCarthy C, McCann HA, Sugrue DD. Evaluation of patients with diabetes mellitus for coronary artery disease using dobutamine stress echocardiography. Coronary Artery Disease1997;8171-4.

17. Griffin ME, Nikookam K, Teh MM, McCann H, O'Meara NM, Firth RG. Dobutamine stress echocardiography: false positive scans in proteinuric patients with type 1 diabetes mellitus at high risk of ischemic heart disease. Diabetic Medicine 1998;15:427-30.
18. Hung MJ, Wang CH, Cherng WJ. Can dobutamine stress echocardiography predict cardiac events in nonrevascularized diabetic patients following acute myocardial infarction? Chest 1999;116:1224-32.
19. Bates JR, Sawada SG, Segar DS, Spaedy AJ, Petrovic O, Fineberg NS, Feigenbaum H, Ryan T. Evaluation using dobutamine stress echocardiography in patients with insulin-dependent diabetes mellitus before kidney and/or pancreas transplantation. Am J Cardiol 1996;77:175-9.
20. Danias PG, Ahlberg AW, Clark BA III, Messineo F, Levine MG, McGill CC, Mann A, Clive J, Dougherty JE, Waters DD, Heller GV. Combined assessment of myocardial perfusion and left ventricular function with exercise technetium-99m sestamibi gated single-photon emission computed tomography can differentiate between ischemic and nonischemic dilated cardiomyopathy. Am J Cardiol 1998;82:1253-8.
21. Naka M, Hiramatsu K, Aizawa T, Momose A, Yoshizawa K, Shigematsu S, Ishihara F, Niwa A, Yamada T. Silent myocardial ischemia in patients with non-insulin-dependent diabetes mellitus as judged by treadmill exercise testing and coronary angiography. Am Heart J 1992;123:46-53.
22. Janand-Delenne B, Savin B, Habib G, Bory M, Vague P, Lassmann-Vague V. Silent myocardial ischemia in patients with diabetes. Who to screen. Diabetes Care 1999;22:1396-1400.
23. Nesto RW, Watson FS, Kowalchuk GJ, Zarich SW, Hill T, Lewis SM, Lane S. Silent myocardial ischemia and infarction in diabetics with peripheral vascular disease: assessment by dipyridamole thallium-201 scintigraphy. Am Heart J 1990;120:1073-7.
24. Lane SE, Lewis SM, Pippin JJ, Kosinski EJ, Campbell D, Nesto RW, Hill T. Predictive value of quantitative dipyridamole-thallium scintigraphy in assessing cardiovascular risk after vascular surgery in diabetes mellitus. Am J Cardiol

1989;64:1275-9.

25. Vanzetto G, Halimi S, Hammoud T, Fagret D, Benhamou PY, Cordonnier D, Denis B, Machecourt J. Prediction of cardiovascular events in clinically selected high-risk NIDDM patients. Prognostic value of exercise stress test and thallium-201 single-photon emission computed tomography. Diabetes Care 1999;22:19-26.

26. Zarich SW, Cohen MC, Lane SE, Mittleman MA, Nesto RW, Hill T, Campbell D, Lewis SM. Routine perioperative dipyridamole 201 Tl imaging in diabetic patients undergoing vascular surgery. Diabetes Care 1996;19:355-60.

Management of Hypertension in the Patient with Diabetes Mellitus

James R. Sowers, MD

Abstract

Cardiovascular disease is the major cause of mortality in persons with type 2 diabetes mellitus and many factors contribute to its high prevalence. Hypertension is one such factor. High blood pressure is about twice as frequent in persons with diabetes mellitus as those without the disease. Information from death certificates indicates that hypertension was implicated in 4.4% of deaths coded to diabetes, and diabetes was involved in 10% of deaths coded to hypertension-related disease. Up to 75% of diabetes-related cardiovascular complications may be attributable to hypertension. These observations have contributed to recommendations for more aggressive lowering of blood pressure in particular to less than 130/85 mm Hg in persons with coexistent diabetes and hypertension. The goal of lowering blood pressure in persons with diabetes is to prevent hypertension-associated death and disability. In older persons, the level of blood pressure and the diagnosis of hypertension should be based on multiple blood pressure measurements obtained in a standardized fashion on at least three occasions. Because of the propensity to orthostatic hypotension, standing blood pressures should be measured in patients on each office visit. Further, because of the increased blood pressure variability of these patients, ambulatory blood pressure measurements or home blood pressure monitoring may be valuable. The consensus blood pressure goal in diabetic persons with hypertension is <130/85. Pharmacologic therapy should be initiated along with lifestyle modifications to lower blood pressure to <130/85 in diabetic persons. The National Institutes of Health Consensus Panel recommended four classes of drugs that are effective as first-line, single-agent therapy. Each drug class has potential advantages and disadvantages but combination therapy is usually necessary for adequate blood pressure control.

Rationale for Blood Pressure Surveillance and Management in the Elderly

The incidence of diabetes, particularly type 2 diabetes, as well as the cost of its treatment and complications is increasing at a rapid rate in industrialized, Westernized cultures such as the United States (1-4). The increasing prevalence of diabetes mellitus tracks with increasing aging, obesity and sedentary lifestyles in these populations (1-8). Type 2 diabetes is also more common in minority populations, including Hispanics and African-Americans, whose relative numbers are increasing in the U.S. (2). Long-term complications of diabetes include blindness, end stage renal disease, non-traumatic amputations, and disabling neuropathy (9). However, cardiovascular disease (CVD) accounts for up to 80% of the deaths in persons with type 2 diabetes mellitus (2,9,10-15). Indeed, data from recent studies indicate that age-adjusted relative risk of death due to CV events in persons with type 2 diabetes is three-fold higher than the general population (9-15). A recent population based study shows that CVD mortality among persons with type 2 diabetes without a previous myocardial infarction was 7.5-fold higher than in those without diabetes (11). Furthermore, the incidence of CVD mortality among persons with diabetes who suffered a myocardial infarction was three-fold higher than similar non-diabetic persons (11).

A number of factors contribute to the high prevalence of CVD in persons with type 2 diabetes. These factors include hypertension, dyslipidemia, hyperglycemia, coagulation and endothelial abnormalities as well as hyperinsulinemia and microalbuminuria (2,9-41). Within the Multiple Risk Factor Intervention Trial (MRFIT) (10), more than five thousand diabetics were followed for 12 years and compared to over three hundred and fifty thousand persons without diabetes. The occurrence of CVD death at the 12 year follow-up was approximately three times higher in diabetic men as in their non-diabetic controls, regardless of systolic blood pressure, age, cholesterol, ethnic group or use of tobacco. The MRFIT results indicated that diabetes is a powerful independent risk factor for CVD mortality above the risk attributable to systolic blood pressure, hypercholesterolemia and cigarette use. This study also confirmed that systolic hypertension, elevated cholesterol and cigarette smoking were also independent predictors of mortality in men with and without diabetes. The presence of one or more of these risk factors had a greater impact on increasing CVD morbidity and mortality in persons with diabetes than in non-diabetics.

Type 2 diabetes is associated with a relatively greater risk for CVD among women than men, and women constitute the majority of the elderly population that is particularly predisposed to development of diabetes (2). Diabetes negates the normal gender difference in the prevalence of CVD (2,42); when adjusted for other risk factors, the risk ratio for increased mortality is 2.4 for diabetic men and 3.5 for women with diabetes mellitus (2,42). Mechanisms by which diabetes overcomes the CV protective effects of estrogen are poorly understood, but likely include effects of hyperglycemia, insulin resistance/hyperinsulinemia, dyslipidemia, platelet abnormalities, coagulation and fibrinolytic dysfunction and oxidative stress/redox alterations and generalized abnormalities of endothelial function (2).

Obesity, especially central obesity, plays an important role in the increased prevalence of both diabetes and hypertension in Westernized, industrialized societies (2,8,20) (Table 4.1). Visceral fat, which is present in omental and paraintestinal sites, is an especially strong risk factor for the development of diabetes, hypertension, insulin resistance/hyperinsulinemia, dyslipidemia and premature coronary artery disease (8). The dyslipidemia associated with visceral obesity, which is also seen in persons with diabetes, is characterized by low levels of HDL cholesterol, high triglyceride levels and a phenotypic small dense LDL particle (8). Concentrations of plasminogen activator inhibitor (PAI-1) are increased in association with visceral obesity, and these increased

Table 4.1

Metabolic and cardiovascular risk factors associated with visceral obesity
■ Insulin resistance
■ Hyperinsulinemia
■ Low HDL-cholesterol
■ High triglyceride levels
■ Elevated Apo lipoprotein B levels
■ Small, dense LDL-cholesterol
■ Elevated fibrinogen levels
■ Elevated plasminogen activator inhibitor
■ Elevated inhibitor – C-reactive protein
■ Elevated systolic and diastolic blood pressure
■ Increased blood viscosity
■ Increased left ventricular hypertrophy
■ Premature atherosclerosis (coronary heart disease and stroke)

concentrations of PAI-1 lead to increased propensity to thrombosis (8). Thus, visceral obesity is often the underlying factor predisposing persons to diabetes and hypertension and associated CVD risk (Table 4.1).

As noted, the dyslipidemia seen in persons with diabetes is characterized by low HDL, high triglycerides and small dense LDL particles (Table 4.2). This dyslipidemia in diabetes is associated with a worse prognosis than in an isolated increase in LDL cholesterol and is more difficult to treat (32). Further, reduction in LDL cholesterol in diabetic persons is associated with at least as great a reduction in CVD risk as seen in persons without diabetes (30-32). For example, subgroup analysis of the Scandinavian Simvastatin Survival Study (4S) trial in a cohort of 201 type 2 diabetic patients suggested that the absolute CVD risk reduction was greater in the diabetic cohort than in the non-diabetic group (30). Subgroup analysis of the Cholesterol and Recurrent Events (CARE) study (31) also showed similar results.

Table 4.2

Lipid, coagulation and fibrinolytic findings in hypertension and diabetes
■ Increased plasma levels of VLDL, LDL and Lp(a) ■ Decreased plasma HDL cholesterol ■ Elevated plasma levels of factor VII and VIII ■ Increased fibrinogen and PAI-1 levels ■ Elevated thrombin – antithrombin complexes ■ Decreased antithrombin III, protein C and S levels ■ Decreased plasminogen activators and fibrinolytic activity ■ Increased endothelial expression of adhesion molecules

Thus, type 2 diabetic patients are at the same risk as non-diabetics who have had a MI or stroke, and have greater atherogenic LDL particles (small, dense, oxidized, glycated, etc.). Therefore, it is recognized that LDL concentration should be lowered in diabetic patients to levels less than 100 mg/dl (32).

Dysfunction of the vascular endothelium plays an important role in the increased propensity to CVD in persons with diabetes and hypertension (2,16). Enhanced oxidative stress and increased production of oxygen free radicals results in increased destruction of vascular nitric oxide (NO), a potent vasodilator (43-45).

Platelet aggregation and adhesion to endothelial cells is increased in persons with hypertension and diabetes (2,16). As it may require higher doses of aspirin to interfere with the endothelial adhesion process, patients with diabetes and hypertension should receive 325 mg of aspirin daily (46) unless an absolute contraindication exists. Blood pressure control is extremely important if aspirin is to be given. In concert with this recommendation, data from the antiplatelet trialists collaboration (47) indicated that the greatest reduction in CVD was achieved with a dose between 165 and 325 mg/day for high risk patients such as those with diabetes and hypertension.

Treatment of Hypertension Associated with Diabetes

Rigorous blood pressure lowering in persons with diabetes and hypertension is necessary to prevent the hypertension-associated death and disability in this population (16). In this regard, hypertension in patients with diabetes often manifests certain unique and challenging characteristics. For instance, many persons with type 2 diabetes lose the normal nocturnal drop in blood pressure (5,16), which may reflect both autonomic dysfunction and abnormal renal-neural sensing of volume/pressure states (48,49). Accordingly, a blood pressure taken during the day time often does not reflect the true pressure load imposed on the cardiovascular system and kidneys. Further, disproportionate elevations of nocturnal blood pressures, especially systolic pressures, may increase CVD risk as well as progression of renal disease in these patients (50). Supine hypertension

Table 4.3

Lifestyle modifications for hypertension prevention and management
■ Lose weight, if overweight ■ Limit alcohol intake to no more than 1 oz (30 ml) of ethanol, e.g., 24 oz of beer, 10 oz of wine or 2 oz of 100 proof whiskey per day, or 0.5 oz of ethanol per day for women and lighter-weight people ■ Increased aerobic physical activity (30-45 minutes most days of the week) ■ Reduce sodium intake to no more than 100 mmol/d (2.4 g of sodium or 6 g of sodium chloride) ■ Maintain adequate intake of dietary potassium (approximately 90 mmol/d) ■ Maintain adequate intake of dietary calcium and magnesium for general health ■ Stop smoking and reduce intake of dietary saturated and cholesterol for overall cardiovascular health

with orthostatic hypotension is relatively common in diabetic patients with autonomic neuropathy (5,16,49,50). Both systolic and diastolic blood pressures are often more labile in persons with diabetic nephropathy, necessitating more measurements (5,16). Finally, renal disease, which occurs in approximately 20% of persons with type 2 diabetes and one third of those with type 1 diabetes is an important promoter of the progression of hypertension in these patients (5,16).

Therapy in patients with hypertension and diabetes should begin with lifestyle modifications (Table 4.3) involving weight reduction, increased physical activity and moderation of salt and alcohol intake (19,20). If goal blood pressure of 130/85 mm Hg is not reached, then pharmacological intervention is indicated (19). Based on clinical trial results, four classes of drugs are effective and appropriate first-line therapy in these patients (Fig. 4.1). Most diabetic patients will require the use of several different agents to achieve a therapeutic goal below 130/85 mm Hg (19,51). Often a low-dose diuretic is needed as part of the therapeutic regimen in order to accomplish goal blood pressures (Fig. 4.1).

ACE inhibitors have been recognized as the first-line antihypertensive therapy in diabetic persons with proteinuria (19,20). Further, as proteinuria is a harbinger for CVD as well as renal disease (17,18), these agents may also afford unique benefits in preventing CVD as well as diabetic nephropathy. Indeed, a cardioprotective effect of ACE inhibitors was suggested from the results of the Appropriate Blood

Figure 4.1

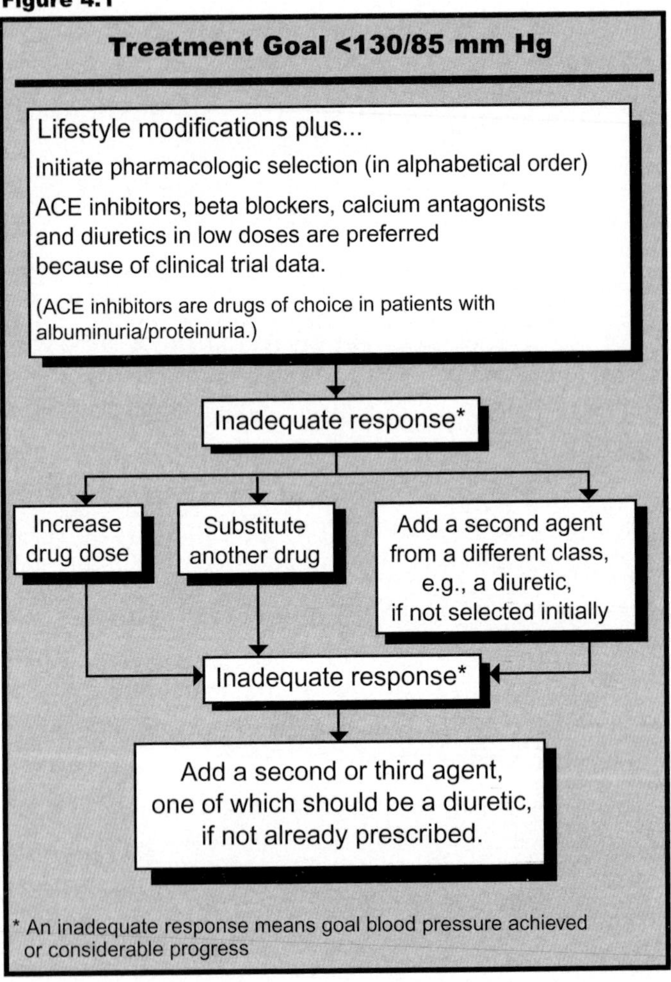

Treatment Goal <130/85 mm Hg
Lifestyle modifications plus...
Initiate pharmacologic selection (in alphabetical order)
ACE inhibitors, beta blockers, calcium antagonists and diuretics in low doses are preferred because of clinical trial data.
(ACE inhibitors are drugs of choice in patients with albuminuria/proteinuria.)
Inadequate response*
Increase drug dose
Substitute another drug
Add a second agent from a different class, e.g., a diuretic, if not selected initially
Inadequate response*
Add a second or third agent, one of which should be a diuretic, if not already prescribed.
* An inadequate response means goal blood pressure achieved or considerable progress

Pressure Control in Diabetes (ABCD) Trial (52). However, in the recent United Kingdom Prospective Diabetes Study (UKPDS) Group report (53,54), blood pressure lowering with an atenolol based program was similarly effective as a captopril based regimen in reducing the incidence of diabetic complications (both microvascular and macrovascular). Many of these patients required both of these drugs plus a diuretic for "tight control of 144/82 mm Hg." In those patients assigned to less tight control (154/87 mm Hg), there was less use of more than one antihypertensive agent. Reductions in risk in the group assigned to tight blood pressure control were 24% in diabetes-related end points, 32% in deaths related to diabetes, 44% in strokes, and 37% in microvascular end points, especially diabetic retinopathy. These results suggest that combination therapy based on either an ACE inhibitor or a beta blocker are very effective in reducing macrovascular and microvascular events as long as blood pressure is adequately lowered. Results of the Fosinopril versus Amlodipine Cardiovascular Events Trial (FACET) suggest that the combination of an ACE inhibitor and a calcium antagonist may be beneficial in reducing CVD in patients with type 2 diabetes and hypertension (55,56). This open label, single center trial was designed to compare the effects of fosinopril and amlodipine on serum lipids and diabetic glycemic control. Subjects were randomly assigned to treatment with either fosinopril or Amlodipine, and if blood pressure was not controlled, the other drug was added. The incidence of CVD events was less in the fosinopril than in the amlodipine treatment groups but the incidence was least in the group that received both antihypertensive agents (56) (Fig. 4.2). These data suggest that addition of a calcium antagonist to baseline ACE inhibitor therapy is a good strategy for treatment of hypertension in this high risk population but that ACE inhibitors may be more beneficial than a calcium channel blocker as initial therapy.

Thiazide diuretics, in relatively low doses, i.e., 25 mg or less of hydrochlorothiazide or chlorthalidone daily, are effective and safe antihypertensive agents in type

Figure 4.2

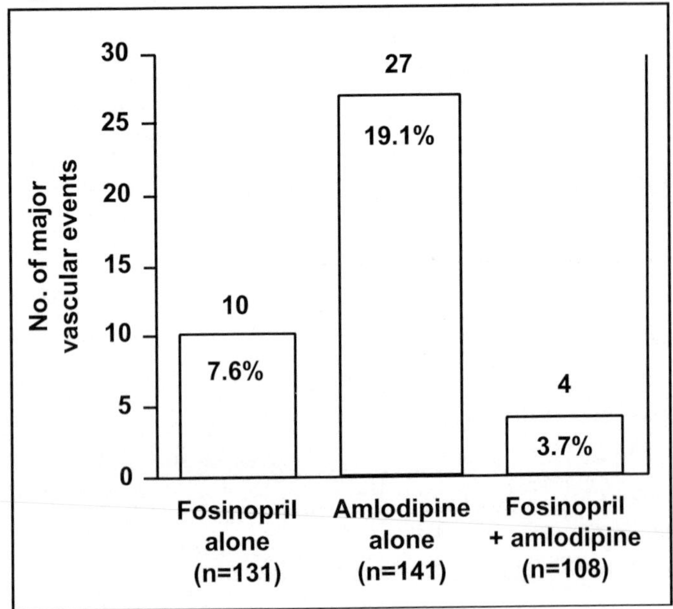

2 diabetic patients (19,20). In the Systolic Hypertension in the Elderly Program (SHEP) study, elderly men with type 2 diabetes derived at least as much benefit, in terms of stroke and coronary heart disease reduction, as those without diabetes (57). Diuretics in low doses are not associated with significant metabolic abnormalities (19,20). Use of diuretics in conjunction with ACE inhibitors usually produces substantial synergism in reducing blood pressure, and use of these agents together further minimizes potential metabolic problems. Diuretics are often a necessary component of the antihypertensive regimen in diabetic patients because of the salt sensitivity and expanded plasma volume that is often present in these patients (5,16,19). This attention to sodium is particularly relevant as several drugs are often required to control blood pressure to levels of <130/85 in these patients.

Results from the subset analysis of type 2 diabetics in the Hypertension Optimal Treatment (HOT) trial (58) suggest that further reduction in diastolic blood pressure below 85 mm Hg is beneficial. The special benefits of aggressive blood pressure lowering in the diabetic population was observed in a recent sub-analysis of this cohort in the Sys-Eur Trial (59). In this trial, while systolic blood pressure was reduced by a comparable amount in each group (–22 ± 16 mm Hg, non-diabetic vs. –22.1 ± 14 mm Hg, diabetic group), the risk reduction in mortality from CVD was 13% for the non-diabetics and 76% for the diabetic patients (59). Thus, the benefit conferred per mm Hg blood pressure reduction appears to be greater in persons with type 2 diabetes than in those with hypertension but without coexistent diabetes mellitus. Moreover, as observed in the UKPDS trial (53,54), the relative benefit on CVD risk reduction is conferred in a far more powerful fashion by intensive blood pressure reduction versus intensive blood glucose control (53). Nevertheless, tight blood glucose control appears important in diabetic patients with coexistent hypertension. The UKPDS demonstrated that sustained reduction of hemoglobin A_{1c} levels (from 7.9% in the conventionally treated patients; 7% in the group receiving intensive care) over a median follow-up of 10 years resulted in a 25% reduction in microvascular complications (proteinuria, retinopathy, etc.) and an overall reduction of diabetes-related events by 12% (60). Results of this study corroborated data from three prospective population-based studies, one from Germany extending 11 years and two from Finland, one of which extended over 10 years (61-63). These prospective studies demonstrate a linear association between coronary artery disease and glycemia in elderly and middle-aged persons with type 2 diabetes. These data emphasize the importance of management of all risk factors in this high risk population.

Summary

Hypertension and type 2 diabetes frequently coexist and pose a major threat of CVD to these patients.

Abundant data have demonstrated a drastic decrease in CVD events if blood pressure is lowered by antihypertensive medications. Goal blood pressure should be set lower than in non-diabetics, i.e., to <130/85 mm Hg. Most diabetic hypertensive patients require more than one medication to lower blood pressure to these goals.

References:

1. Amos AF, McCarty DJ, Zemel P. The rising global burden of diabetes and its complications: estimates and projections to the year 2010. Diab Med 1997;14(Suppl 5):S1-S5.
2. Sowers JR. Diabetes mellitus and cardiovascular disease in women. Arch Intern Med 1998;158:617-621.
3. Muggeo M, Verlate G, Bonora E, et al. The Verona Diabetes Study: a population based survey on known diabetes mellitus prevalence and 5-year all cause mortality. Diabetologia 1995;38(3):318-325.
4. Berger M, Jorgens V, Flatten G. Healthcare for persons with non-insulin dependent diabetes mellitus. The German experience. Ann Int Med 1996;124(Suppl):153-155.
5. Sowers JR, Farrow SL. Treatment of elderly hypertensive patients with diabetes, renal disease and coronary heart disease. Am J Geriatr Cardiol 1996;5:57-70.
6. Mykkünen L, Küsiste J, Pyorala K, Laakso M, Hofner SM. Increased risk of non-insulin dependent diabetes in elderly hypertensive subjects. J Hypertens 1994;2:1425-1432.
7. Flegal KM, Caroll MD, Kuczarski RJ, Johnson CL. Overweight and obesity in the United States: Prevalence and trends, 1960-1994. Int J Obes Relat Metab Disord 1998;22(1):39-47.
8. Sowers JR. Obesity and cardiovascular disease. Clin Chem 1998;44(8):1821-1825.
9. Klein R. Hyperglycemia and microvascular and macrovascular disease in diabetes. Diabetes Care 1995;18(2): 258-268.

10. Stamler J, Vaccaro O, Neaton JD, Wentworth D. Diabetes, other risk factors and 12-year cardiovascular mortality for men screened in the Multiple Risk Factor Intervention Trial. Diabetes Care 1993;263(17):2335-2340.

11. Haffner SM, Lehto S, Ronnemma T, Pyorala K, Laakso M. Mortality from coronary heart disease in subjects with type 2 diabetes and in non-diabetic subjects with and without myocardial infarction. N Engl J Med 1998;339(4):229-234.

12. Abraira C, Colwell J, Nuttall F, Sawin CT, Henderson W, Comstock JP, et al (Veterans Affairs Cooperative Study on Glycemic Control and Complications in Type II Diabetes [VACSDM] Group). Cardiovascular events and correlates in the Veterans Affairs diabetes feasibility trial. Arch Intern Med 1997;157:181-188.

13. Lehto S, Ronnemaa T, Haffner SM, Pyorala K, Kallio V, Laakso M. dyslipidemia and hyperglycemic predict coronary heart disease events in middle-aged patients with NIDDM. Diabetes 1997;48:1354-9.

14. Wei M, Gaskil SP, Haffner SM, Stern MP. Effects of diabetes and level of glycemia on all-cause and cardiovascular mortality: The San Antonio Heart Study. Diabetes Care 1998;21(7):1167-77.

15. Hanefeld M, Fischer S, Julius U, Schulze J, Schwanebeck U, Schmechel H, Ziegelasch HJ, Lindner J. Risk factors for myocardial infarction and death in newly detected NIDDM: the Diabetes Intervention Study, 11-year follow-up. Diabetologia 1996;39(12):1577-1583.

16. Sowers JR, Epstein M. Diabetes mellitus and associated hypertension, vascular disease and nephropathy: An update. Hypertension 1995;26:869-879.

17. Kuusisto J, Mykkanen L, Pyorala K, et al. Hyperinsulinemia and microalbuminuria: a new risk indicator for coronary heart disease. Circulation 1995;90:831.

18. Dinneen SF, Gerstein HC. The association of micro- albuminuria and mortality in non-insulin-dependent diabetes mellitus. A systematic overview of the literature. Arch Intern Med 1997;157:1413-1418.

19. National High Blood Pressure Education Program Working Group report on hypertension in diabetes. Hypertension 1994;23:145-158.
20. Sixth Report of the Joint National Committee on Detection, Evaluation and Treatment of High Blood Pressure (JNC-VI). Arch Intern Med 1997;157:2413-2446.
21. Chen JW, Jen SL, Lee WL, Hsu NW, Lin SJ, Ting CT, Chang MS, Wang PH. Differential glucose tolerance in dipper and nondipper essential hypertension. Diabetes Care 1998;21(10):1743-1748.
22. Peles E, Goldstein DS, Akselrod S, Nitzan H, Azaria M, Almog S, Dolphin D, Halkin H, Modan M. Interrelationships among measures of autonomic activity and cardiovascular risk factors during orthostasis and the oral glucose tolerance test. Clin Auton Res 1995;5:271-278.
23. UKPDS Group. UK Prospective Diabetes Study 38: Tight blood pressure control and risk of macrovascular and microvascular complications in type 2 diabetes. BMJ 1998;317:703-713.
24. UK prospective Diabetes Study (UKPDS) Group. Intensive blood-glucose control with sulphonylureas or insulin compared with conventional treatment and risk of complications in patients with type 2 diabetes (UKPDS 33). Lancet 1998;352:837-853.
25. Uusitupa MI, Niskanen LK, Siitonen O, Voutilainen E, Pyorala K. Ten-year cardiovascular mortality in relation to risk factors and abnormalities in lipoprotein composition in type 2 (non-insulin-dependent) diabetic and non-diabetic subjects. Diabetologia 1993;36(11):1175-1184.
26. Kuusisto J, Mykkanen L, Pyorala K, Laakso M. NIDDM and its metabolic control predict coronary heart disease in elderly subjects. Diabetes 1994;43(8):960-967.
27. Laakso M. Glycemic control and risk of coronary heart disease in patients with NIDDM: the Finnish studies. Ann Intern Med 1998;124:127-130.

28. UK Prospective Diabetes Study (UKPDS) Group. Effect of intensive blood-glucose control with metformin on complications in overweight patients with type 2 diabetes (UKPDS 34). Lancet 1998;352:854-865.
29. Jeppesen J, Hein HO, Suadicani P, Gyntelberg F. Triglyceride concentration and ischemic heart disease: an eight-year follow-up in the Copenhagen Male Study. Circulation 1998;97(11):1029-1036.
30. Pyorala K, Pedersen TR, Kjekshus J, Faergeman O, Olsson AG, Thorgeirsson G. Cholesterol lowering with simvastatin improves prognosis of diabetic patients with coronary heart disease. A subgroup analysis of the Scandinavian Simvastatin Survival Study (4S). Diabetes Care 1997;20(4):614-620.
31. Sacks FM, Pfeffer MA, Moye LA, Rouleau JL, Rutherford JD, Cole TG, Brown L, Warnica JW, Aranold JM, Wun CC, Davis BR, Braunwald E. The effect of pravastatin on coronary events after myocardial infarction in patients with average cholesterol levels. Cholesterol and Recurrent Events Trial investigators. N Engl J Med 1996;335(14):1001-1009.
32. American Diabetes Association. Management of dyslipidemia in adults with diabetes. Diabetes Care 1998; 21:179-182.
33. UKPDS Group. Efficacy of atenolol and captopril in reducing risk of macrovascular and microvascular complications in type 2 diabetes. UKPDS 39. BMJ 1998;317:713-720.
34. Tatti P, Pahor M, Byington RP, DiMauro P, Guaresco R, Strollo G, Strotts F. Outcome results of the Fosinopril versus Amlodipine Cardiovascular Events Randomized Trial (FACET) in patients with hypertension and NIDDM. Diabetes Care 1998;21:579-603.
35. Sowers JR. Comorbidity of hypertension and diabetes: the Fosinopril versus Amlodipine Cardiovascular Events Trial (FACET). Am J Cardiol 1998;82:15R-19R.
36. Staussen JA, Fagard R, Thys L, et al. For the Systolic Hypertension-Europe (Syst-Eur) trial investigators. Morbidity and mortality in the placebo-controlled European trial on isolated systolic hypertension in the elderly. Lancet 1997;350:757-764.

37. Curb JD, Pressel MS, Cutler JA, Applegate WB, et al. Effect of a diuretic-based antihypertensive treatment on cardiovascular disease risk in older diabetic patients with isolated hypertension. JAMA 1996;276:1886-1892.

38. Bakris GL. Progression of diabetic nephropathy. A focus on arterial pressure level and methods of reduction. Diabetes Res Clin Pract 1998;39:S35-S42.

39. Hansson L, Zanchetti A, Carruthers S, et al for the HOT Study Group. Effects of intensive blood pressure-lowering and low-dose aspirin in patients with hypertension: principal results of the Hypertension Optimal Treatment (HOT) randomized trial. Lancet 1998;351:1755-1762.

40. Curb JD, Pressel SL, Cutler JA, Savage PJ, Applegate WB, Black H, Camel G, Davis BR, Frost PH, Gonzalez N, Guthrie G, Oberman A, Rutan GH, Stamler J. Effect of diuretic-based antihypertensive treatment on cardiov ascular disease risk in older diabetic patients with isolated systolic hypertension. Systolic Hypertension in the Elderly Program Cooperative Research Group. JAMA 1996;276(23):1886-1892.

41. Tuomilehto J, Rastenyte D, Birkenhager WH, Thijs L, Antikainen RI, Bulpitt CJ, et al for the Systolic Hypertension in Europe Trial Investigators. Effects of calcium channel blockers in older patients with diabetes and systolic hypertension. N Eng J Med 1999;340: 677-684.

42. Garcia MJ, McNamara PM, Gordon T, Kannel WB. Morbidity and mortality in diabetes in the Framingham population: sixteen-year follow-up study. Diabetes 1990;13:631-654.

43. Consentino F, Hishikawa K, Kutusic C, Luscher TF. High glucose increases nitric oxide synthase expression and superoxide anion generation in human aortic endothelial cells. Circulation 1997;96:25-28.

44. Muniyappa R, Srinivas PR, Ram J, Sowers JR. Calcium and protein kinase C mediate high glucose-induced inhibition of inducible nitric oxide synthase in vascular smooth muscle cells. Hypertension 1998;31:289-295.

45. Griendling K, Masuko UF. WADH/NADPH oxidase and vascular function. Trends in Cardiovasc Med 1997;7: 301-307.

46. American Diabetes Association. Aspirin therapy in diabetes. Diabetes Care 1998;21(suppl):45-46.

47. Antiplatelet Trialists Collaboration. Collaborative overrun of randomized trials of antiplatelet therapy-1: prevention of death, myocardial infarction, and stroke by prolonged antiplatelet therapy in various categories of patients. BMJ 1994;308:81-106.

48. Chen JW, Jen SL, Lee WL, Hsu NW, Lin SJ, Ting CT, Chang MS, Wang PH. Differential glucose tolerance in dipper and nondipper essential hypertension. Diabetes Care 1998;21(10):1743-1748.

49. Peles E, Goldstein DS, Akselrod S, Nitzan H, Azaria M, Almog S, Dolphin D, Halkin H, Modan M. Interrelationships among measures of autonomic activity and cardiovascular risk factors during orthostasis and the oral glucose tolerance test. Clin Auton Res 1995;5:271-278.

50. Sowers JR, Farrow SL. Treatment of elderly hypertensive patients with diabetes, renal disease and coronary heart disease. Am J Geriatr Cardiol 1996;5:57-70.

51. Bakris GL. Progression of diabetic nephropathy. A focus on arterial pressure level and methods of reduction. Diabetes Res Clin Pract 1998;39:S35-S42.

52. Estacio RO, Schrier RW Antihypertensive therapy in type 2 diabetes: implications of the appropriate blood pressure control in diabetes (ABCD) trial. Am J Cardiol 1998; 12(9B):9R-14R.

53. UKPDS Group. UK Prospective Diabetes Study 38: Tight blood pressure control and risk of macrovascular and microvascular complications in type 2 diabetes. BMJ 1998;317:703-713.

54. UKPDS Group. Efficacy of atenolol and captopril in reducing risk of macrovascular and microvascular complications in type 2 diabetes. UKPDS 39. BMJ 1998;317:713-720.

55. Tatti P, Pahor M, Byington RP, DiMauro P, Guaresco R, Strollo G, Strotts F. Outcome results of the Fosinopril versus Amlodipine Cardiovascular Events Randomized Trial (FACET) in patients with hypertension and NIDDM. Diabetes Care 1998;21:579-603.
56. Sowers JR. Comorbidity of hypertension and diabetes: the Fosinopril versus Amlodipine Cardiovascular Events Trial (FACET). Am J Cardiol 1998;82:15R-19R.
57. Curb JD, Pressel MS, Cutler JA, Applegate WB, et al. Effect of a diuretic-based antihypertensive treatment on cardiovascular disease risk in older diabetic patients with isolated hypertension. JAMA 1996;276:1886-1892.
58. UK Prospective Diabetes Study Group. Tight blood pressure control and risk of macrovascular and microvascular complications in type 2 diabetes: UKPDS 38. BMJ 1998;317:703-713.
59. Hansson L, Zanchetti A,Carruthers SB, Dahlof B, Elmfeldt D, Julius S, Menard J, Rahn KH, Wedel H, Westerling S. Effects of intensive blood pressure-lowering and low-dose aspirin in patients with hypertension: principal results of the Hypertension Optimal Treatment (HOT) randomized trial. HOT Study Group. Lancet 1998;351:1755-1762.
60. UK Prospective Diabetes Study Group. Intensive blood-glucose control with sulphonylureas or insulin compared with conventional treatment and risk of complications in patients with type 2 diabetes (UKPDS 33). Lancet 1998;352:837-853.
61. Uusitupa MI, Niskanen LK, Siitonen O, Voutilainen E, Pyorala K. Ten-year cardiovascular mortality in relation to risk factors and abnormalities in lipoprotein composition in type 2 (non-insulin-dependent) diabetic and non-diabetic subjects. Diabetologia 1993;36(11):1175-1184.
62. Kuusisto J, Mykkanen L, Pyorala K, Laakso M. NIDDM and its metabolic control predict coronary heart disease in elderly subjects. Diabetes 1994;43(8):960-967.
63. Hanefeld M, Fischer S, Julius U, Schulze J, Schwanebeck U, Schmechel H, Ziegelasch HJ, Lindner J. Risk factors for myocardial infarction and death in newly detected NIDDM: the Diabetes Intervention Study, 11-year follow-up. Diabetologia 1996;39(12):1577-1583.

Lipid Disturbances: Diagnosis and Treatment in the Patient with Diabetes Mellitus

Alan Chait, MD

Atherosclerotic cardiovascular disease is the major cause of morbidity and mortality in the United States in diabetes, especially type 2. Type 2 diabetic subjects without previous clinical coronary artery disease have the same risk of dying of coronary disease as non-diabetic subjects with who have had a previous myocardial infarction (Fig. 5.1). The increased cardiovascular disease risk in diabetes is contributed to by the clustering of cardiovascular risk factors (1). These include hypertension, dyslipidemia, hyper-

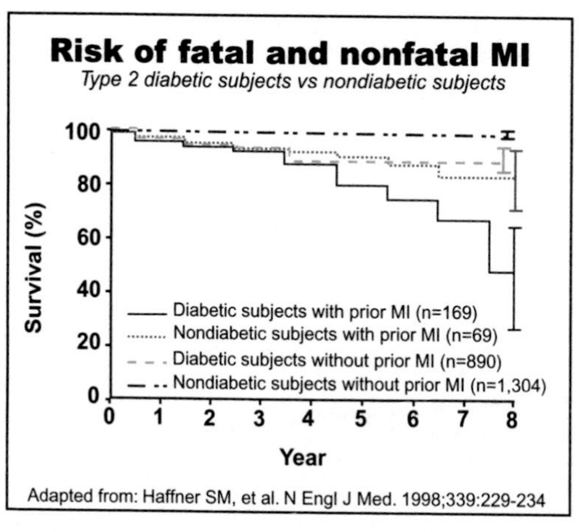

Figure 5.1. Increased probability of death from coronary disease in diabetes. Kaplan-Meier estimates the probability of death from coronary heart disease in 1,059 subjects with type 2 diabetes and 1,378 non-diabetic subjects with and without prior myocardial infarction. MI denotes myocardial infarction. I bars indicate 95% confidence intervals.

insulinemia, hyperglycemia, central obesity and hemostatic risk factors such as hyperfibrinogenemia and an increase in the level of plasminogen activator-1.

The dyslipidemia that so frequently occurs in diabetes increases cardiovascular risk. Further, lipid-lowering therapy markedly reduces the risk of cardiovascular disease. Hence, an approach to the diagnosis and management of diabetic dyslipidemia is a critical component in the management of the patient with diabetes.

What is Diabetic Dyslipidemia?

Diabetic dyslipidemia refers to a constellation of abnormalities of plasma lipids and lipoproteins characterized by hypertriglyceridemia, low levels of high density lipoprotein (HDL) cholesterol, and the presence of small, dense low density lipoprotein (LDL) particles (Table 5.1). The magnitude of elevation of plasma triglycerides, and the extent of HDL reduction often is quite mild. LDL-cholesterol levels tend to be towards the high end of the normal range, or only modestly elevated.

Table 5.1

Features of diabetic dyslipidemia
■ Mild to modest fasting hypertriglyceridemia
■ Increased postprandial lipoproteins
■ Accumulation of remnants of the triglyceride-rich lipoproteins
■ Small, dense LDL
■ LDL levels high normal or only mildly elevated
■ Modest decrease in HDL-cholesterol

Assessment of plasma lipoproteins using research techniques demonstrates the presence of an increase in dense very low density lipoprotein (VLDL) particles, an accumulation of remnant lipoproteins in the intermediate density lipoprotein (IDL) range, the presence of small, dense LDL, a reduction in HDL particles, with compositional abnormalities in HDL, and the loss of a subset of HDL_2 particles (2). There also is an increase in post-prandial lipoproteins, to which the artery wall is exposed for much of the day. These compositional changes are not detected by the routine measurement of plasma lipids and lipoproteins, as performed in the clinical laboratory. Routine lipid and lipoprotein analysis usually detects mild to modest abnormalities in triglycerides and HDL-cholesterol.

Workup of the Diabetic Patient

The workup should include assessment of whether the patient has type 1 or type 2 diabetes, since the cardiovascular disease risk is much greater in type 2 diabetes. The increased risk in type 2 diabetes is likely to be contributed to by the clustering of cardiovascular risk factors, which should be sought in the individual patient. These risk factors also coexist in the central obesity/insulin resistance syndrome, even in the absence of frank hyperglycemia. These patients may have impaired fasting glucose levels. The patient also should be evaluated for complications of diabetes. It is particularly important to evaluate for the presence of nephropathy, including assessment of microalbuminuria. Nephropathy markedly increases cardiovascular disease risk, including in type 1 diabetes.

A personal history of previous cardiovascular disease should be sought. Current assessments may include evaluation by a cardiologist and non-invasive assessment for coronary artery disease. However, because of the poor outcome in patients with diabetes even in the absence of clinical cardiovascular disease, some experts believe that all patients with type 2 diabetes should be treated as if they have established atherosclerotic disease. A careful family history should be obtained for evidence of premature vascular disease, dyslipidemia and diabetes.

It clearly is not feasible to perform the above-mentioned sophisticated lipid and lipoprotein techniques during the routine management of all diabetic patients. From a clinical standpoint, it usually will suffice to measure plasma cholesterol, triglycerides, and LDL and HDL

Table 5.2

Workup for diabetic dyslipidemia
Type of diabetes — type 1 vs. 2 vs. impaired fasting glucose
Other cardiovascular risk factors
Complications of diabetes
Renal incl. microalbuminuria
Autonomic neuropathy
Personal history of cardiovascular disease
(? cardiology evaluation, incl. EKG, stress test, stress ECHO)
Family history
Lipid profile
Plasma cholesterol, triglyceride, LDL-cholesterol, HDL-cholesterol
Apoplipoprotein B

cholesterol. However, abnormalities in these measures, even if mild, signify the presence of the marked compositional changes that have been discussed earlier. Diabetic dyslipidemia, however mild, should be taken seriously because of its association with a markedly increased risk of cardiovascular disease. Measurement of plasma apo B levels, where available, gives an indication of the number of atherogenic lipoprotein particles, since there is one molecule of apo B per particle in the VLDL, IDL and LDL density range. Plasma apo B levels frequently are elevated in diabetes. The routine evaluation of newer cardiovascular risk factors such as Lp(a), homocysteine and C-reactive protein are not currently recommended.

Based on careful workup of the patient according to this scheme, it is possible to stratify the patient into moderate or high risk categories (Table 5.3).

Consequences of Diabetic Dyslipidemia

The major consequence of diabetic dyslipidemia is an increased risk of atherosclerotic complications. The

Table 5.3

Risk stratification in adults with diabetes
Moderate risk
LDL < 130 mg/dl, no other risk factors
Type 1, no other risk factors, no nephropathy
High risk
Established cardiovascular disease
LDL > 130 mg/dl
Positive family history of premature vascular disease
Presence of other cardiovascular risk factors

presence of dyslipidemia in diabetes increases the already high risk of cardiovascular disease by about 2-4 fold (3). In the insulin resistance syndrome and type 2 diabetes, other risk factors tend to cluster with dyslipidemia. This clustering of risk factors is associated with a markedly increased risk of cardiovascular disease. Interestingly, non-diabetic family members of individuals with diabetic dyslipidemia also have an increased cardiovascular risk. This observation suggests that these relatives may have inherited the insulin resistance/central obesity syndrome, in which there is a clustering of cardiovascular risk factors, yet may not have developed full-blown diabetes. This observation may also explain the "ticking-clock" hypothesis, which states that the clock starts ticking for the development of microvascular complications at the time of the onset of hyperglycemia, whereas the beginning of the development of macrovascular complications can precede the onset of clinical diabetes by many years (4). It has been suggested that the existence of dyslipidemia and other risk factors associated with the insulin resistance/central obesity syndrome prior to the onset of hyperglycemia, in part, explains why so many diabetic patients already have coronary artery disease at the time of the diagnosis of their diabetes.

There are multiple mechanisms whereby diabetic dyslipidemia may accelerate atherosclerosis by interaction with the artery wall (Fig. 5.2). It currently is believed that matrix molecules, particularly proteoglycans, can retain lipoproteins that enter the subendothelial space. Once retained, the lipoproteins can undergo oxidative modification, which greatly increases their atherogenicity. Lipoprotein retention and oxidation is believed to be increased in diabetes, which may in part explain the increased risk in this disorder. Small, dense LDL can enter the subendothelial space more

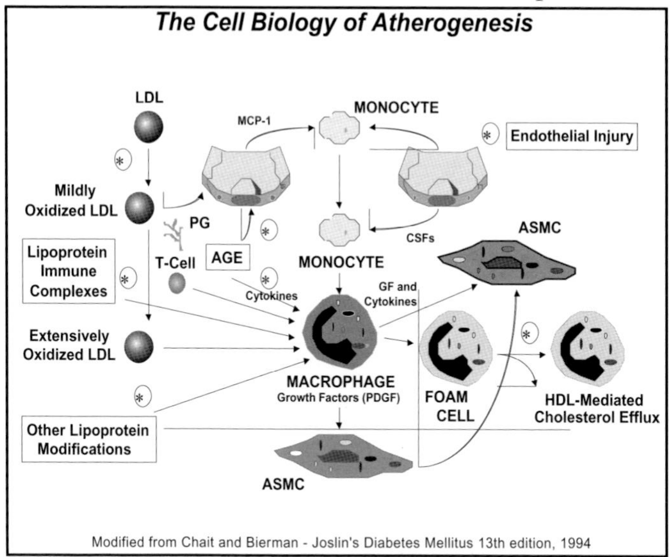

Figure 5.2. The role of diabetes in the pathogenesis of atherosclerosis. Apo B-containing lipoproteins cross the endothelial barrier (EC) and are retained in the subendothelial space by proteoglycans (PG). After undergoing oxidation, the oxidized lipoproteins stimulate the adhesion, chemotaxis and differentiation of macrophages, and the uptake of oxidized lipoproteins by macrophage scavenger receptors. Lipoproteins also modulate the expression of growth factors and cytokines secreted by smooth muscle cells that have migrated to the intima from the media. They also can affect the expression of tissue factor and plasminogen activator inhibitor-1 (PAI-1), which can lead to plaque rupture and thrombosis. An "*" designates all of the processes that can be increased in diabetes.

readily than larger more buoyant LDL particles. Also, small, dense LDL binds better than more buoyant LDL to proteoglycans and also are more readily oxidized. In addition, small, dense LDL are present as part of an atherogenic lipoprotein phenotype, in which many other atherogenic lipoproteins accumulate in plasma (2). In addition, low levels of HDL can result in impaired cholesterol efflux from the artery wall.

The autoxidation of glucose is associated with the generation of oxygen free radicals. This oxidant stress can regulate a number of oxidation sensitive genes that play a role in atherogenesis. In addition, glucose autoxidation can facilitate the oxidation of LDL with all its consequences. The formation of advanced glycation end products (AGE) can interfere with the function of key proteins and can induce intracellular oxidant stress. AGE-lipoproteins can be formed, which have many biological properties similar to that of oxidized LDL. Although there is a relationship between indices of glycemic control and macrovascular disease end points, this relationship is far less strong than that between glycemic control and microvascular disease (5).

Table 5.4

Lifestyle modification in diabetes
■ Diet ■ Weight control ■ Decrease saturated fat and dietary cholesterol ■ Replace with CHO or monosaturated fat ■ Regular exercise program

Management of Diabetic Dyslipidemia

Most patients with type 2 diabetes are overweight or have central obesity. Since many of the cardiovascular risk factors that are associated with the insulin resistance syndrome and type 2 diabetes improve with weight loss, i.e., dyslipidemia, hypertension, hyperinsulinemia and insulin resistance, hyperglycemia, and central obesity, a program designed to achieve weight control is highly desirable. However, the ability to maintain weight loss is seldom effective in the long term. Such a program should include regular physical exercise, which appears to help sustain weight loss.

All patients with diabetic dyslipidemia should be on a diet that is low in saturated fat and cholesterol. There is considerable controversy as to whether to replace a portion of the reduced saturated fat calories with carbohydrates, monounsaturated or polyunsaturated fat. Isocaloric replacement of saturated fat with carbohydrate may increase plasma triglyceride levels in susceptible individuals. Therefore, triglycerides should be monitored in diabetic subjects consuming very high carbohydrate diets, particularly if they are gaining weight. The use of very low carbohydrate, high protein diets is of concern, since they tend to be high in saturated fat, which can increase the risk of cardiovascular disease. Although many patients report initial success with weight loss on these diets, they have not been shown to be successful in achieving sustained weight loss over time.

Drug Therapy

Fibrates

The use of lipid-lowering drugs has been shown to reduce cardiovascular end points in patients with diabetes in post-hoc analysis of those trials in which sufficiently large numbers of diabetic subjects have been included to allow for reasonable analysis (Table 5.5). Only one primary prevention trial using fibrates has performed a post-hoc

Table 5.5

Clinical trials of lipid-lowering drugs in diabetic subgroups				
Study	***Drug***	***# diabetic subjects***	***% ↓ in controls***	***% ↓ in diabetics***
Fibrate Trials – 1° Prevention				
Helsinki	Gemfibrozil	135	34	60
Fibrate Trials – 2° Prevention				
VA-HIT	Gemfibrozil	620	24	24
Statin Trials – 1° Prevention				
AFCAPS/ TexCAPS	Lovastatin	155	37	42
Statin Trials – 2° Prevention				
4S	Simvastatin	202	32	55
CARE	Pravastatin	586	23	25
LIPID	Pravastatin	792	25	19

analysis on diabetic patients. In the Helsinki Heart Study, a large percent reduction in cardiovascular end points was observed in diabetic subjects who took gemfibrozil relative to controls (6). However, because of the small number of diabetic subjects in this study, this effect was not statistically significant (Fig. 5.3). The Veterans Affairs Cooperative Studies Program High Density Lipoprotein Intervention Trial (VA-HIT) was a secondary prevention study that used gemfibrozil in patients with low HDL, high triglycerides and relatively normal LDL levels (7). About 25% of the study subjects had diabetes. Those with diabetes benefited from gemfibrozil to a similar extent as those without diabetes. Since fibrates lower triglycerides and increase HDL levels, these effects are perhaps not

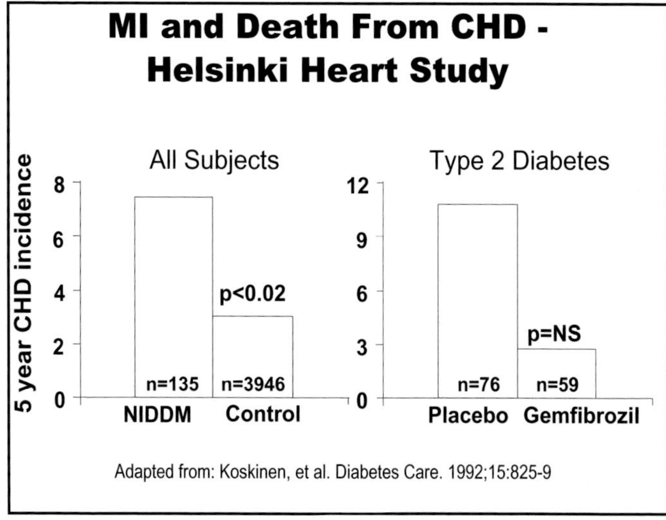

Figure 5.3. Subgroup analysis in diabetic subjects in the Helsinki Heart Study. In the Helsinki Heart Study, gemfibrozil reduced CHD events, but the results were not statistically significant because of the small number of events in this primary prevention trial and because of the small number of diabetic subjects.

surprising. More studies currently are underway to specifically test the effect of fibrates in reducing cardiovascular disease consequences in diabetes.

Statins

Even though elevations of LDL are not a major component of diabetic dyslipidemia, statins, whose primary effect is to lower LDL cholesterol, also have been shown to be effective in reducing cardiovascular disease in diabetes. The only primary prevention statin trial to

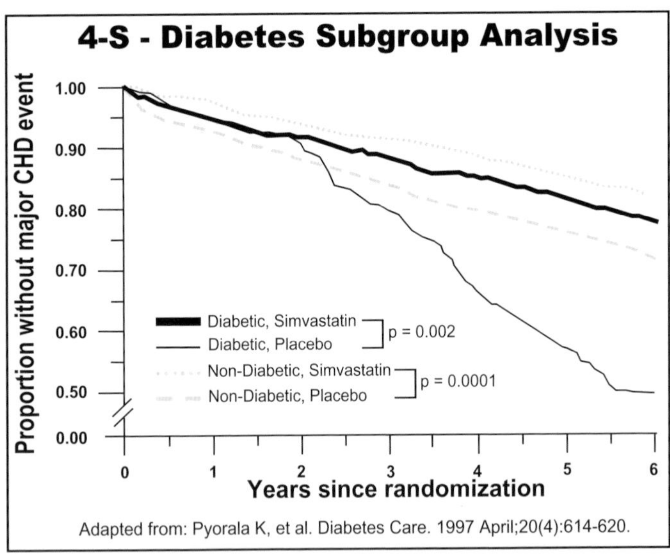

Figure 5.4. Subgroup analysis in diabetic subjects in the Scandinavian Simvastatin Survival Study (4S). In both diabetic and non-diabetic subgroups of 4S (a secondary prevention trial), simvastatin significantly decreased major CHD events (P=0.002). The Kaplan-Meier survival curve for simvastatin-treated diabetic subjects actually lies above that for the placebo group in non-diabetic subjects.

date that has included a diabetic subgroup is the Air Force/Texas Coronary Atherosclerosis Prevention Study (AFCAPS-TexCAPS) (8). In this study, the use of lovastatin in subjects with diabetes had a similar effect to its use in non-diabetic subjects. Several secondary prevention trials have used statins. In the Scandinavian Simvastatin Survival Study (4S), simvastatin use was associated with a greater percent reduction in cardiovascular end-points in subjects with diabetes than in those without diabetes. Again, because of the small number of diabetic subjects in that trial, and because the study was not powered to test the effect of the drug in diabetes per se, these differences between diabetic subjects and controls were not statistically significant. However, the effect of the statin versus placebo was highly significant in the diabetic subgroup (9) (Fig. 5.4). In the Cholesterol and Recurrent Events (CARE) trial, the diabetic subgroup that received pravastatin had a similar reduction in event rate as the group without diabetes (10). In the Long-term Intervention with Pravastatin in Ischemic Disease (LIPID) trial, lovastatin therapy was associated with a slightly lower decrease in event rate in the diabetic versus the non-diabetic group (11). However, again, the use of a statin led to a reduction in event rate relative to the use of a placebo.

These post-hoc analyses showed that use of a statin had at least as good an effect in the diabetic subgroups as in those without diabetes. Since the number of events in diabetic subjects is far greater than in non-diabetic controls, the absolute benefit to be accrued by treating patients with diabetes with a statin is impressive. Trials that focus specifically on diabetic subjects, including primary prevention trials, are ongoing at present. Thus, even though the primary abnormality is not an elevation of LDL-cholesterol, reduction of LDL levels by statins may play an important role in the management of diabetic dyslipidemia. An alternate explanation for the beneficial effect of the statins is that they also might reduce the levels of other atherogenic lipoprotein particles. At present, statins appear to be the drugs of choice for the treatment of diabetic dyslipidemia, unless the triglyceride levels are very elevated, in which case it is reasonable to start treatment with a fibrate.

Combination therapy

Frequently, optimal lipoprotein levels are not achieved with either class of drug alone, in which case combination therapy, using both a statin and a fibrate may be tried. For example, if plasma triglyceride levels remain elevated with the use of a statin, a fibrate may be added. Conversely, if LDL levels are unacceptably high after the use of a fibrate alone, or if LDL levels increase as they often do with fibrate therapy, the addition of a statin may be considered. The frequency of myopathy is increased with the combined use of a stain and fibrate, especially in the presence of renal failure. For this reason, combination therapy is somewhat controversial. This complication should be watched for carefully with the use of combination therapy. Studies are ongoing to evaluate the effect of this combination of lipid lowering drugs in diabetes, and to evaluate the extent of myopathy that occurs with combination therapy. The Lipid and Diabetes Study being performed in Europe should provide useful information regarding the relative benefits of statins versus fibrates as monotherapy, and about the safety of combination therapy.

The American Diabetes Association has provided guidelines (12) for the use of lipid-lowering therapy in patients with diabetes (Table 5.6). These guidelines apply particularly to individuals with type 2 diabetes.

Treatment decisions are based on LDL cholesterol levels in adults with diabetes. For diabetic patients with multiple CHD risk factors [low HDL (<35 mg/dl), hypertension, smoking, family history of CVD, or microalbuminuria or proteinuria], some authorities recommend initiation of drug therapy when LDL levels are between 100 and 130 mg/dl.

Table 5.6

Therapeutic decision for lipid-lowering therapy in adults with diabetes

	Nutritional therapy		***Drug therapy***	
	Initiation level	***LDL goal***	***Initiation level***	***LDL goal***
With CHD, PVD or CVD	> 100 mg/dl	≤ 100 mg/dl	> 100 mg/dl	≤ 100 mg/dl
Without CHD, PVC, or CVD	> 100 mg/dl	≤ 100 mg/dl	≥ 130 mg/dl*	≤ 100 mg/dl

* For diabetic patients with multiple CHD risk factors [low HDL (< 35 mg/dl), hypertension, smoking, family history of CVD, or microalbuminuria or proteinuria], some authorities recommend initiatin of drug therapy when levels are between 100 and 130 mg/dl.

A suggested algorithm for the use of drugs is shown in Table 5.7. The starting drug is based on the magnitude of the triglyceride elevation. Because more information is available regarding the statins, they usually are the drugs of choice, unless the triglyceride levels are very high (e.g. >400 mg/dl). The use of a fibrate as the starting drug is reasonable at triglyceride levels above 400 mg/dl. These recommendations might change when the results of several ongoing studies become available.

Although niacin decreases plasma triglyceride and LDL-cholesterol and increases HDL-cholesterol levels, it also worsens insulin resistance and glycemic control in diabetes. Therefore, it is relatively contraindicated in diabetes. It may however occasionally be used with caution, but usually requires more intensive therapy for glycemic control. Bile acid binding resins tend to increase plasma triglyceride levels, and therefore have little place in the management of diabetic dyslipidemia.

Since dyslipidemia in diabetes usually occurs in association with other cardiovascular risk factors, such as hypertension, aggressive blood pressure management should be pursued concurrently. Studies discussed elsewhere in this primer point out the importance of blood pressure control in diabetes. Due to the frequent association of abnormalities of coagulation in this setting, aspirin, which appears to benefit the patient with diabetes in a similar manner to non-diabetic subjects, should be used unless otherwise contraindicated. The

Table 5.7

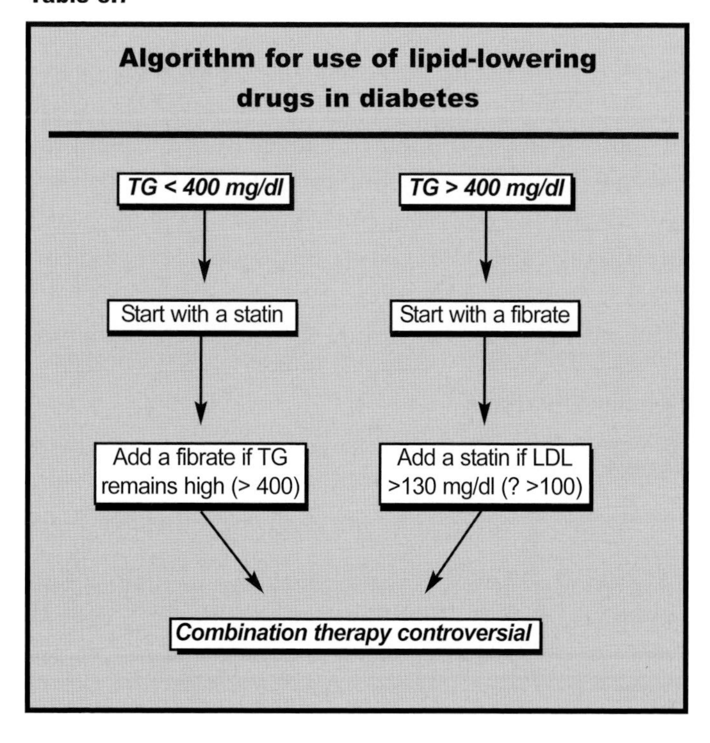

Algorithm for use of lipid-lowering drugs in diabetes
TG < 400 mg/dl
TG > 400 mg/dl
Start with a statin
Start with a fibrate
Add a fibrate if TG remains high (> 400)
Add a statin if LDL >130 mg/dl (? >100)
Combination therapy controversial

role of glycemic control in the prevention and treatment of macrovascular disease in diabetes remains less clear than the clear-cut benefits of aggressive treatment of lipids and blood pressure. However, tight glycemic control plays a critical role in prevention of the microvascular complications of diabetes, and should be undertaken vigorously.

Other strategies to reduce macrovascular complications await further investigation. For example, the use of antioxidants to inhibit oxidative stress and lipoprotein oxidation makes theoretical sense, but awaits testing in placebo controlled clinical trials. Also, drugs that specifically raise HDL levels are under development. With time they might prove useful, since low levels of HDL are an important feature of diabetic dyslipidemia.

Special Situations

Type 1 Diabetes

The risk of cardiovascular disease is somewhat lower in type 1 diabetes than in type 2, except in the presence of nephropathy. In addition, most type 1

Table 5.8

Type 1 diabetes
■ Do not usually have the features of insulin resistance
■ HDL-cholesterol usually normal or even increased
■ LDL goals should be higher (≤130 mg/dl), unless secondary prevention (≤100 mg/dl), other risk factors or nephropathy
■ Ensure adequate nutrition for optimal growth and development

patients do not have features of the insulin resistance syndrome with its constellation of associated risk factors (Table 5.8). Further, HDL levels tend to be normal or even elevated in most treated type 1 patients. Therefore, a less aggressive approach to the management of diabetic dyslipidemia seems reasonable in type 1 diabetes. In particular, a target LDL-cholesterol of <100 mg/dl is probably lower than required for all type 1 patients, especially those that are young. A LDL-cholesterol goal of <130 mg/dl seems reasonable for most type 1 patients, unless they have established atherosclerotic disease, nephropathy or other cardiovascular risk factors, in which the goal for LDL-cholesterol should be <100 mg/dl.

Chylomicronemia Syndrome

On rare occasions plasma triglyceride levels exceed 2000 mg/dl. When triglyceride levels are this high, patients can have clinical features of the chylomicronemia syndrome (Table 5.9).

Triglyceride levels of this magnitude usually occur

Table 5.9

Features of the Chylomicronemia Syndrome
■ Abdominal pain/pancreatitis ■ Eruptive xanthomata ■ Memory loss and decreased mentation ■ Dysesthesias
Can occur when triglyceride levels > 2000 mg/dl

in type 2 rather than type 1 diabetes, and usually are the result of the co-existence of diabetes (or the insulin resistance syndrome) and a common familial form of hypertriglyceridemia. A primary goal of therapy is to reduce triglyceride levels to prevent pancreatitis. The drug of choice for this purpose is a fibrate. Other secondary forms of hypertriglyceridemia such as hypothyroidism should be treated, and drugs that raise triglyceride levels, such as alcohol, estrogens, glucocorticoids, diuretics and beta blockers should be replaced or eliminated, if possible. However, these individuals also are at an increased risk of cardiovascular disease and may require statins to reduce their LDL levels, in addition to therapy for their marked hypertriglyceridemia.

References:

1. Haffner SM, Valdez RA, Hazuda HP, Mitchell BD, Morales PA and Stern MP: Prospective analysis of the insulin-resistance syndrome (syndrome X). Diabetes 41:715-22, 1992.
2. Chait A and Brunzell JD: Diabetes, Lipids, and Atherosclerosis, in Diabetes Mellitus: A Fundamental and Clinical Text, D. LeRoith, S.I. Taylor, and J.M. Olefsky, Editors. Lippincott-Raven: Philadelphia. p. 772-780, 1996.
3. Chait A and Haffner S: Diabetes, Lipids and Atherosclerosis, in Endocrinology (in press), L.J. DeGroot and J.L. Jameson, Editors. W.B. Saunders, 2000.
4. Haffner SM, Stern MP, Hazuda HP, Mitchell BD and Patterson JK: Cardiovascular risk factors in confirmed prediabetic individuals: Does the clock for coronary heart disease start ticking before the onset of clinical diabetes? JAMA 263:2893-2898, 1990.

5. Turner RC, Millns H, Neil HA, Stratton IM, Manley SE, Matthews DR and Holman RR: Risk factors for coronary artery disease in non-insulin dependent diabetes mellitus: United Kingdom Prospective Diabetes Study (UKPDS: 23). Br Med J 316:823-8, 1998.
6. Koskinen P, Mänttäri M, Manninen V, Huttunen J and Heinonon O: Coronary heart disease incidence in NIDDM patients in the Helsinki Heart Study. Diabetes Care 15:825-829, 1992.
7. Rubins HB, Robins SJ, Collins D, Fye CL, Anderson JW, Elam MB, Faas FH, Linares E, Schaefer EJ, Schectman G, Wilt TJ and Wittes J: Gemfibrozil for the secondary prevention of coronary heart disease in men with low levels of high-density lipoprotein cholesterol. Veterans Affairs High-Density Lipoprotein Cholesterol Intervention Trial Study Group. N Engl J Med 341:410-8, 1999.
8. Downs JR, Clearfield M, Weis S, Whitney E, Shapiro DR, Beere PA, Langendorfer A, Stein EA, Kruyer W and Gotto AM, Jr.: Primary prevention of acute coronary events with lovastatin in men and women with average cholesterol levels: results of AFCAPS/TexCAPS. Air Force/Texas Coronary Atherosclerosis Prevention Study. JAMA 279:1615-22, 1998.
9. Pyörälä K, Pedersen TR, Kjekshus J, Faergeman O, Olsson AG and Thorgeirsson G: Cholesterol lowering with simvastatin improves prognosis of diabetic patients with coronary heart disease. A subgroup analysis of the Scandinavian Simvastatin Survival Study (4S). Diabetes Care 20:614-20, 1997.
10. Goldberg RB, Mellies MJ, Sacks FM, Moye LA, Howard BV, Howard WJ, Davis BR, Cole TG, Pfeffer MA and Braunwald E: Cardiovascular events and their reduction with pravastatin in diabetic and glucose-intolerant myocardial infarction survivors with average cholesterol levels: subgroup analyses in the cholesterol and recurrent events (CARE) trial. The Care Investigators. Circulation 98:2513-9, 1998.

11. The Long-Term Intervention with Pravastatin in Ischaemic Disease (LIPID) Study Group: Prevention of cardiovascular events and death with pravastatin in patients with coronary heart disease and a broad range of initial cholesterol levels. N Engl J Med 339:1349-1357, 1998.

12. American Diabetes Association Position Statement: Management of dyslipidemia in adults with diabetes. Diabetes Care 23:557-562, 2000.

Prevention and Management of Renal Disease in the Patient with Diabetes Mellitus

George L. Bakris, MD

Introduction

Hypertension is defined by the Joint National Committee Report VI (JNC VI) as an arterial pressure of >140/90 mm Hg for the general population (1). The goal blood pressure, however, for those with diabetes is <130/85 mm Hg as defined by the 1997 JNC VI criteria and as <130/80 mm Hg defined by the 1999 Canadian Hypertension Society and the 2000 consensus report of the National Kidney Foundation (2,3).

It is important to note, however, that only 27% of all non-elderly people with a diagnosis of hypertension are controlled to levels <140/90 mm Hg (1). Moreover, if we include those over the age of 65 years and those at high risk (those with diabetes and renal insufficiency) who require blood pressure reduction to <130/80 mm Hg, <3% are controlled. Poor blood pressure control may have contributed to a flattening of the previously declining cardiovascular mortality rates associated with hypertension treatment. Moreover, this degree of blood pressure reduction has never had an effect on the incidence of renal failure in the United States (Fig. 6.1) (4).

Both unilateral and bilateral renal parenchymal disease can cause hypertension. Chronic renal parenchymal disease of various etiologies is the most common secondary cause of arterial hypertension, accounting for about 50 to 60 % of all secondary causes of hypertension (5). Hypertension is a major risk factor, among individuals with renal parenchymal disease; it predicts who will ultimately develop end stage renal disease (ESRD). Moreover, poorly controlled hypertension in such individuals will hasten the decline in renal function.

Hypertension is also present in over 80% of people with type 2 diabetes and about 35 to 40% of people with type 1 diabetes. Its presence clearly identifies people who will develop ESRD related to diabetes (6,7). Possible reasons for this impact of elevated arterial pressure on the vasculature as well as the kidney, in a person with diabetes,

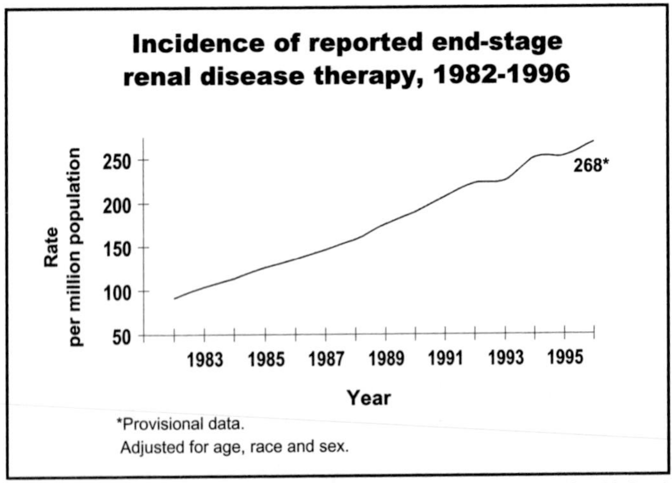

Figure 6.1. The incidence of endstage renal disease in the United States up to 1997. Data from USRDS, 1999.

may be secondary to further increases in already stimulated cytokines such as the interleukins, transforming growth factor-β (TGFβ) endothelin and others (8). Thus, the presence of elevated arterial pressure in a diabetic is like adding gasoline to an already burning fire.

Unlike the normal kidney, the nephrons of a diabetic kidney are not able to accommodate large fluctuations in arterial pressure; thus they have lost their ability to autoregulate (Fig. 6.2) (9). This is very important to

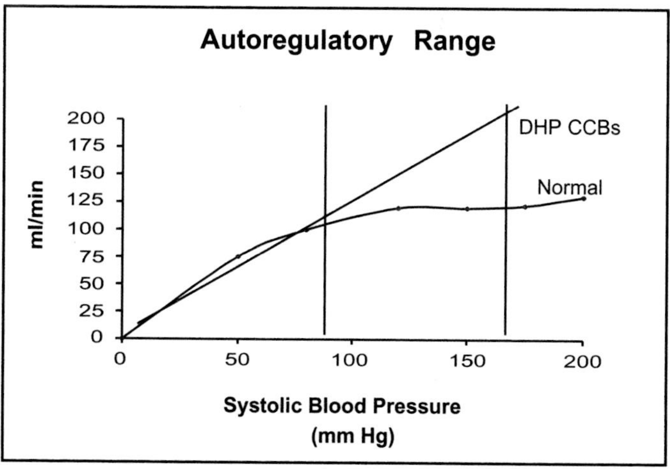

Figure 6.2. The relationship between a range of blood pressure levels and glomerular filtration rate and/or renal blood flow to the kidney. Under normal circumstances renal function remains relatively stable over a wide range of blood pressures (> 90 mm Hg <180 mm Hg, systolic). Above or below these ranges, renal function becomes totally dependent on systemic pressure. Loss of autoregulation either pharmacologically induced, as with dihydropyridine CCBs or disease-induced, as in diabetes, transposes the physiologically appropriate sigmoidal relationship between these variables to a linear one. Thus, it requires a much lower blood pressure in order to maintain renal function at a more physiological level, i.e., GFR, 110-120 ml/min in some with normal renal function at baseline.

consider when a goal blood pressure is determined and antihypertensive therapy to achieve this goal is being prescribed.

As in the diabetic patient, hypertension development in non-diabetic renal disease accompanies progressive renal failure and, if uncontrolled, hastens the decline of renal function. This latter observation is exemplified in an analysis of the Modification of Dietary Protein in Renal Disease trial (MDRD). In this trial more than 80% of patients with renal failure had hypertension, an association that correlated positively with the degree of pre-existing renal insufficiency (10).

Hypertension due to renal parenchymal disease usually occurs in the presence of bilateral rather than unilateral kidney disease. The mechanisms that generate elevation in blood pressure in most of these cases relate to volume overload and altered sodium homeostasis. Additionally, areas of intrarenal ischemia lead to activation of neurohumoral systems, i.e., the renin-angiotensin-aldosterone system and the sympathetic nervous system that also contribute to increases in blood pressure.

Regardless of the etiology, it is likely that blood pressure reduction to levels of <130/80 mm Hg in those with renal disease and diabetes reduces cardiovascular disease risk and renal disease progression. Moreover, those with renal disease and greater than one gram per day of proteinuria require even lower levels of arterial pressure, i.e., <125/75 mm Hg in order to maximally slow renal disease progression (2,10).

This chapter will review the trials that generated the data establishing that lower levels of blood pressure are required to best preserve renal function. It will also provide a method for achieving the recommended goals.

Evidence for Lower Blood Pressure Goals

The MDRD trial was the first to randomize and assess the impact of different levels of blood pressure control in patients with renal insufficiency and proteinuria, largely from non-diabetic causes. Patients randomized to a mean arterial pressure of <92 mm Hg manifested significantly slower rates of decline in renal function than those randomized to mean pressures between 102-106 mm Hg (10). Moreover, the subgroup of African-Americans randomized to the lower blood pressure in this trial had far better renal outcomes. The question, however, as to whether further reductions in blood pressure will optimally slow or stop progression of renal disease in African-Americans will be definitively answered by the ongoing African-American Study of Kidney Disease (AASK) trial due to be completed in 2002 (11).

The observation that lower levels of blood pressure are associated with maximal slowing of renal disease progression is also seen in a post hoc analysis of the Multiple Risk Factor Intervention Trial (MRFIT). In this trial of over 330,000 people with hypertension, the relative risk for development of ESRD started to rise significantly when the average blood pressure rose above 127/82 mm Hg (12).

A lower level of blood pressure control is also recommended for those with diabetic renal disease. Evidence from post hoc analyses of prospective studies in diabetic nephropathy as well as meta-analyses supports the notion that arterial pressure must be reduced to levels well below 130/85 mm Hg to maximally slow or prevent progression of nephropathy (Fig. 6.3). A summary of the JNC VI recommendations that define both the level to which blood pressure should be reduced as well as those in whom these recommendations apply is presented in Table 6.1. The National Kidney Foundation recommendation for blood pressure goal to maximally slow diabetic nephropathy is <130/80 mm Hg,

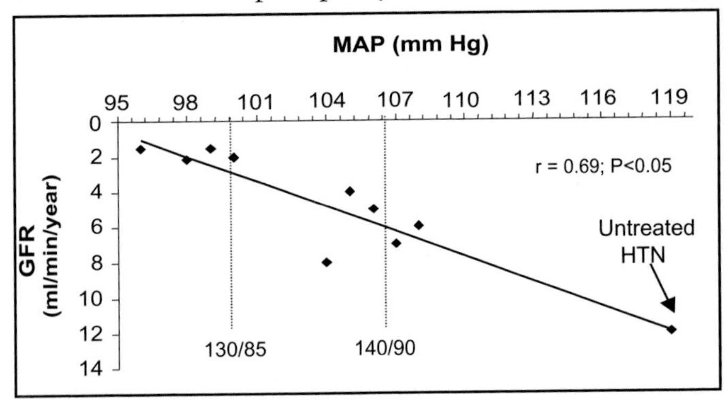

Figure 6.3. A summary of clinical trials, each >3 years duration, in diabetic and non-diabetic persons with pre-existing renal insufficiency. This analysis demonstrates the importance of the degree of blood pressure reduction in relation to decline in renal function over time. One reason for requiring lower blood pressures in order to slow renal disease progression may relate to the loss of autoregulatory ability of the kidney in such patients. Adapted from reference 32

a level congruent with the recommendation of the Canadian Hypertension Society but lower than the JNC VI recommendation of <130/85 mm Hg (2,3). A paradigm for how to achieve this goal is discussed later in the text.

Table 6.1

Recommendations of drug therapy intervention for people with hypertension and co-morbid conditions

Blood pressure stages	*Systolic or diastolic*	*Risk stratification*	*Plan*
Pressure			
High normal	130-139 or 85-89	Diabetes, heart failure, renal disease ±TOD/CCD*	Drug therapy
Stage – 1	140-159 or 90-99	Failure of lifestyle modification for 6-12 months with one risk factor or diabetes, heart failure renal disease ±TOD/CCD*	Drug therapy
Stage – 2 & 3	≥160 or ≥100	Diagnosis made by 2 or more readings at 2 or more visits after an initial screening	Drug therapy

* TOD – target organ damage
CCD – clinical cardiovascular disease (includes: LVH, angina, prior myocardial infarction or coronary revascularization, congestive heart failure, stroke, transient ischemic attack, nephropathy, peripheral arterial disease, retinopathy)
Risk factors – smoking, dyslipidemia, diabetes mellitus, age >60 years, male sex or postmenopausal female, family history of cardiovascular disease

Lastly, no discussion about blood pressure level would be complete without a discussion of the J curve. Since its inception in 1979, the concept that reducing diastolic blood pressure to levels below 85 mm Hg is associated with a paradoxical increase in cardiovascular mortality has been controversial. It is clear, however, that a J curve exists among patients with established symptomatic coronary artery disease, unstable angina or those who are in the immediate post myocardial infarction period. A post hoc analysis of clinical trials that have randomized to different levels of blood pressure, the MDRD trial, the Hypertension Optimal Treatment trial and the Appropriate Blood Pressure Control in Diabetes (ABCD) trial, demonstrates no significant increase in cardiovascular events among those with renal insufficiency, proteinuria and diastolic blood pressures of >75 but <85 mm Hg (10,13,14). Moreover, in the high risk group of diabetics, a higher cardiovascular event rate at a diastolic blood pressure goal of <85 mm Hg was not seen in the United Kingdom Prospective Diabetes Study (UKPDS) (15). Thus, in the absence of any clear evidence of coronary disease or unstable angina, "high risk" patients such as African-Americans and those with diabetes or renal insufficiency should have their blood pressures brought to the recommended goal <130/80 mm Hg.

Given this background it is important that a physician have a logical and methodical approach to the treatment of hypertension. This chapter presents the approach to the treatment of hypertension in persons with diabetes endorsed by the National Kidney Foundation in 2000. This approach is predicated on many of the guidelines put forth in the Joint National Committee Report (JNC VI).

Treatment of the Hypertensive Patient

Adequate assessment and management of the hypertensive patient begins by obtaining a concise medical history and by proper measurement of blood pressure. Evaluation of patients with hypertension has three objectives: first, to identify known causes of high blood pressure; secondly, to assess the presence or absence of target organ damage and cardiovascular disease, the extent of the disease and the response to therapy; and lastly, to identify other cardiovascular risk factors or concomitant disorders that may define prognosis and guide treatment.

Selection of Initial Drug Therapy

Selection of an initial antihypertensive agent as well as an add-on antihypertensive medication for a given patient depends upon many factors including a risk factor profile (smoking, obesity, etc.), and presence of co-morbid conditions (asthma, gout, etc.) in a diabetic patient. Some factors to consider before initiation of monotherapy are summarized in Table 6.2.

Table 6.2

Factors to consider before selection of monotherapy in a hypertensive patient

Factor	*Useful*	*Not useful or unsafe*
Hyperkalemia	ARBs, non-DHPCCBs, diuretic, α blocker	ACEI, β blockers
Renal failure* (GFR ≤30)	non-DHPCCBs, loop-active diuretic, ?ACEI, ?ARB	High dose ACEI
Nephrotic syndrome	ACEI with non-DHPCCBs or ARBs, ?loop-active diuretic	DHPCCBs, minoxidil, hydralazine, α blockers
Coronary artery disease	ACEI, non-DHPCCBs, β blockers	minoxidil, hydralazine
Autonomic neuropathy	Central α agonists, ?β blockers	α blockers, hydralazine, minoxidil
Microalbuminuria	ARBs, ACEI, CCBs	minoxidil, hydralazine
Side-effect profile	ARBs, ACEI, CCBs, carvedilol	β blockers, high dose diuretics, central α agonists, minoxidil, hydralazine
Peripheral vascular disease	ARBs, ACEI, non-DHPCCBs, α blockers	β blockers

* This population usually needs diuretic therapy in addition to other antihypertensive therapy for edema control.
Carvedilol – α, β blocker. All CCBs increase renal blood flow in early diabetes, which may not be of benefit.
Non-DHPCAs only subclass of CCBs shown to consistently decrease albuminuria.

GFR – glomerular filtration rate; ACEI – angiotensin-converting enzyme inhibitors; Non-DHPCCBs – nondihydropryidine calcium channel blockers; ARBs – angiotensin receptor blockers; Central α agonists – clonidine, methyldopa

An Approach to Achieve Goal Blood Pressure

Diabetic patients, even in the absence of other risk factors, are complicated patients. Their risk of dying from a cardiovascular event, in the absence of any prior history of a myocardial infarction, is similar to non-diabetic patients with a prior history of myocardial infarctions or stroke (16). Moreover, in the presence of co-morbid conditions, such as being elderly or African-American, smoking, dyslipidemia, obesity or surrogate markers of end organ disease such as left ventricular hypertrophy or microalbuminuria, these patients become even more complicated. Co-morbid conditions in patients with hypertension mandate tailoring antihypertensive therapy to optimally reduce cardiovascular risk and renal disease progression. An approach to tailoring antihypertensive therapy to slow or stop renal disease progression in such patients is illustrated in figure 6.4. It will be the focus of discussion for the remainder of the chapter. To put the recommendations in this figure into context we must also examine the renal and cardiovascular impact of certain markers of vascular/endothelial cell disease, namely microalbuminuria.

Microalbuminuria (MA)

MA is defined as spot urine albumin/creatinine ratio of 30 to 299 mg/g. It is a predictor of cardiovascular and renal death in patients with diabetes. A recent retrospective analysis of over 2,000 people followed for

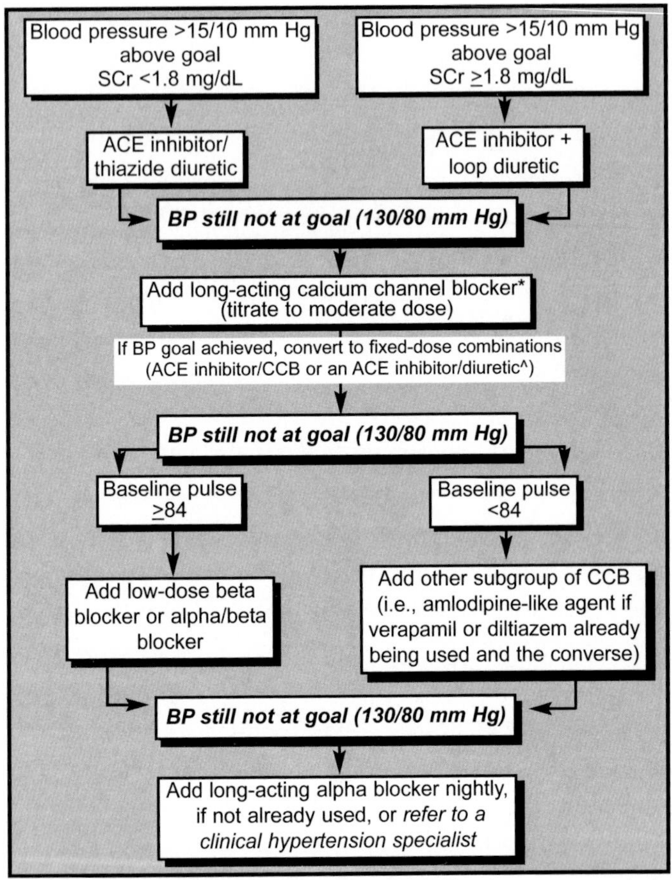

Figure 6.4. A suggested paradigm by which blood pressure goals in people with renal insufficiency and/or diabetes can be achieved by the least intrusive means possible. Everyone with diabetes and/or renal insufficiency should be instructed on lifestyle modifications as per the JNC VI. Everyone, however, should be started on therapy if blood pressure is greater than 130/85 mm Hg * Note: If BP <15/10 mm Hg above goal (130/80 mm Hg) then ACE inhibitor alone may be used. ^ ACE inhibitor should be the same if two different fixed-dose combinations are used. ** Non-dihydropyridine CCBs (verapamil, diltiazem have been shown to reduce both CV mortality and progression of diabetic nephropathy independent of an ACE inhibitor)

ten years demonstrated that presence of MA was second only to smoking for increasing the relative risk of developing ischemic heart disease (Fig. 6.5) (17). Moreover, even if blood pressure was controlled, MA conferred independent risk for CV disease, (Fig. 6.5). MA is a particularly sensitive predictor of cardiovascular risk in all patients, particularly those with diabetes, and the presence of MA is linked to abnormal vascular responsiveness (17). Thus, MA may reflect the history of blood pressure control. In this way it is a type of "HbA_{1c}" indicator of the kidney injury.

A blunted rise or reduction in MA, however, is associated with a slowed progression of renal disease (18-20). The class of antihypertensive medications

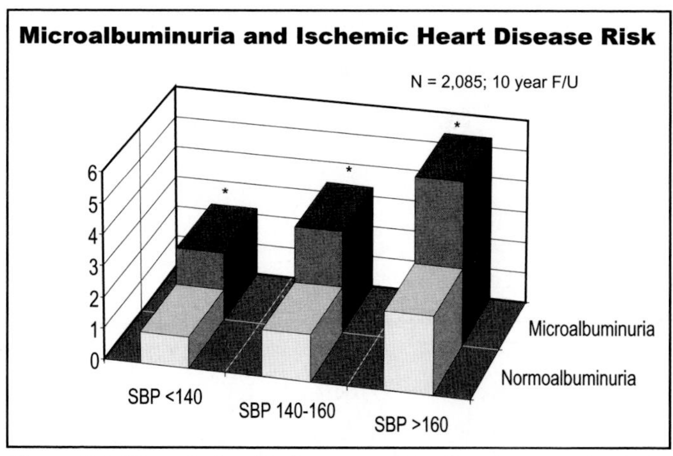

Figure 6.5. The relationship between microalbuminuria and risk for ischemic heart disease. Note that even with blood pressure levels of <140 mm Hg, microalbuminuria still confers a two-fold greater risk of ischemic disease development compared to those who are normoalbuminuric.
* P <0.05 compared to normoalbuminuria

known to most effectively reduce MA is the ACE inhibitors. These agents reduce albuminuria by reducing intraglomerular pressure as well as decreasing glomerular size selectivity. The effects of different classes of antihypertensive agents on MA as well as related metabolic parameters are summarized in Table 6.3.

It should be clear that any agent or group of agents that adequately lowers arterial pressure to levels <130/80 mm Hg will slow progression of nephropathy. From the available clinical data, both ACE inhibitors and non-dihydropyridine calcium antagonists reduce albuminuria individually but together have additive anti-albuminuric effects independent of further reductions in blood pressure (17-26). Additive effects have also been reported with the combination of an ACE inhibitor and angiotensin receptor blocker (27). Moreover, the addition of an ACE inhibitor to a dihydropyridine CCB (amlodipine-like) results in a reduction in albuminuria, an event not seen with the dihydropyridine CCB alone (28). ACE inhibitors are generally well tolerated. Therefore, ACE inhibitors should be first in line for the treatment of hypertension in diabetes and included in all antihypertensive regimens in such patients.

The role of angiotensin receptor blockers for treatment of diabetic nephropathy is unclear at this time. However, animal studies suggest that these agents will be as good as ACE inhibitors in slowing progression of renal disease. This class has a significantly lower incidence of cough and hyperkalemia when compared with an ACE inhibitor.

Table 6.3

Effects of antihypertensive therapy on metabolic, cardiovascular and renal markers associated with increased morbidity and/or mortality in the patient with diabetes and hypertension

	Central α agonists	*α blockers*	*α, β blockers*	*Vasodilator*
Metabolic				
Cholesterol (LDL)	→	→	→	→
Insulin resistance	→	↑	→ ↑	→ ↑
Glucose control	→	→	→	→
Cardiovascular				
LV hypertrophy	↓	↓	↓	→ ↑
Renal/ endothelial fx.				
Microalbuminuria	→	→	→ ↓	→

	β blockers	*ACEI*	*ARBs*	*CAs*	*Diuretics*
Metabolic					
Cholesterol (LDL)	→ * ↑	→	→	→	→ ↑
Insulin resistance	→ ↑	↓	↓	→	→ ↑
Glucose control	→ ↓	→ ↑	→	* ↑ →	→ ↑
Cardiovascular					
LV hypertrophy	↓	↓	↓	↓	→ ↓
Renal/ endothelial fx.					
Microalbuminuria	→ ↓	↓	↓	** → ↓	→ ↓

Note: This table summarizes the general trends in the literature.
HDL – high-density lipoprotein; LDL – low-density lipoprotein; ACEI – ACE Inhibitor; ARB – Angiotensin II receptor antagonist; LV – left ventricular; fx – function; → no effect; ↑ increase; ↓ decrease
* Only β blockers with intrinsic sympathomimetic activity; only when used in high doses, e.g., 480 mg/d diltiazem, 480 mg/d verapamil, 90 mg/d nifedipine
** Only non-dihydropyridine calcium antagonists (CAs, verapamil, diltiazem)

Albuminuria/Renal Dysfunction

Albuminuria is defined as an albumin/creatinine ratio of 300 mg/g or more in a spot urine. From the available data it is clear that aggressive blood pressure reduction (<130/80 mm Hg) is needed to maximally slow progression of renal disease, especially among patients with elevated serum creatinine, >1.4 mg/dl. As previously stated, ACE inhibitors slow progression of diabetic nephropathy to a greater extent than other antihypertensive agents, assuming blood pressure reduction to levels around 140/90 mm Hg. Their effect on progression of non-diabetic renal disease is also excellent, albeit more a function of the level to which blood pressure is reduced. Moreover, ACE inhibitors tend to reverse endothelial dysfunction in the coronary bed (29).

In spite of this evidence from many long-term clinical trials, there is a general concern of clinicians to use ACE inhibitors in such patients. This concern stems from a rise in serum creatinine that follows when the drug is given. While this may be a concern, it should only be worrisome if the serum potassium rises or if the creatinine continues to climb after a month of therapy.

The time sequence and causes of this rise in serum creatinine following ACE inhibitor administration are shown and explained in figure 6.6. It is common to see increases in serum creatinine of up to 30% within one to four months of ACE inhibitor initiation (30); these increases are acceptable starting with a baseline of up to

3 mg/dl (30). Long-term clinical trials have confirmed that this reduction in renal function plateaus within a month. Moreover, after ACE inhibitors were discontinued following ten years of therapy, glomerular filtration rate (GFR) returned to baseline. This return to baseline GFR has not been reported with other classes of antihypertensive agents studied (30).

Thus, while any class of antihypertensive agent may be used to achieve this new recommended lower level of blood pressure to preserve renal function, the following should be kept in mind. First, blood pressure will never be adequately controlled in patients with renal insufficiency without the use of a diuretic, usually

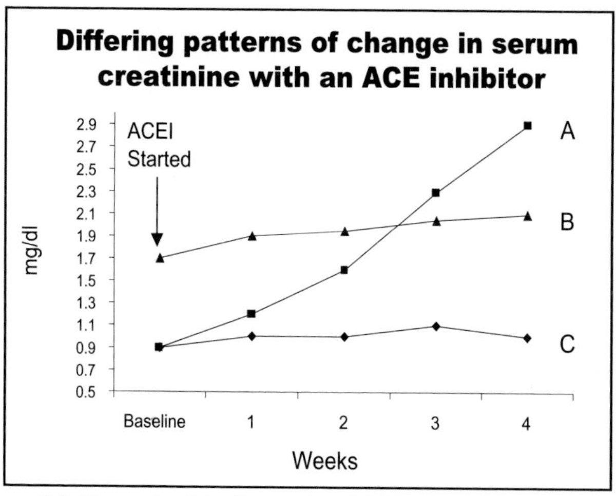

Figure 6.6. The potential effects of an ACE inhibitor on serum creatinine under three separate scenarios:

A – person who is either volume depleted or has heart failure with volume depletion or has bilateral renal artery stenosis.

B – Person with renal insufficiency who is euvolemic.

C – Normal renal function with euvolemia.

a loop diuretic. Secondly, various combinations of medications will be needed to achieve blood pressure reduction. One of these combinations should contain an ACE inhibitor. If side effects are noted with the ACE inhibitor, an angiotensin II receptor blocker may be substituted to ensure renal protection and blood pressure reduction.

Combination Antihypertensive Therapy

It is well known that an agent from a single antihypertensive drug class will only reduce blood pressure to <140/90 mm Hg in 45-50% of individuals with hypertension. This percentage is much lower if people with renal insufficiency or diabetic nephropathy are treated, especially since their goal blood pressure is <130/80 mm Hg. Moreover, data from clinical trials demonstrate that anywhere from an average of 3.5 to 4.2 different antihypertensive medications are required to lower blood pressure to <130/80 mm Hg among patients with renal insufficiency (Fig. 6.7) (31-32). Thus, fixed dose combination therapy provides a way to potentially improve compliance since a person can take the same number of medications in half the pills.

In the early 1960s, fixed-dose combination antihypertensive therapy was introduced with a reserpine/thiazide diuretic combination (31). Since then, there have been many new fixed-dose combinations introduced. Because of their convenient dosing schedule, mostly once daily, these agents are of particular use in "high risk" populations that require aggressive reduction of blood pressure. Table 6.4 illustrates the variety of fixed-dose combinations available for use in the world. It also highlights those approved as first-line therapy for hypertension.

An ideal way to halt the progression of renal disease and better control arterial pressure is to combine two complementary groups of medications. Smaller than the single agent therapeutic doses of two different drugs are combined in a single pill to reduce arterial pressure to the same level that would be achieved by a higher dose of an individual component. In this way they are not only additive for blood pressure reduction, but have fewer side effects. Moreover, many fixed-dose combinations act to counteract each other's side effects.

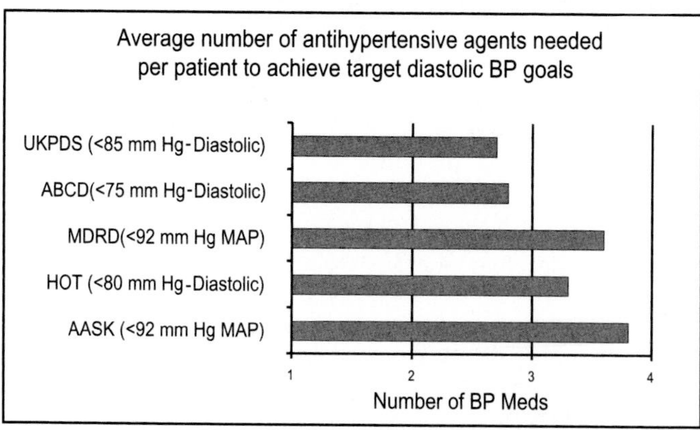

Figure 6.7. A summary of all randomized clinical trials that evaluate the effects of two different blood pressure levels on either cardiovascular outcomes or renal disease progression. Note that in some cases mean arterial pressure is used and in other cases diastolic pressure. Average number of different antihypertensive medications to achieve blood pressure goal is 3.2 different agents.

Table 6.4

Fixed-dose combinations available in the United States	
Drug	***Trade name***
Beta-adrenergic blockers and diuretics	
Atenolol 50 or 100 mg/chlorthalidone, 25 mg	Tenoretic
Bisoprolol fumarate 2.5, 5 or 10 mg/hydrochlorothiazide, 6.25 mg	Ziac*
Metoprolol tartrate 50 or 100 mg/hydrochlorothiazide, 25 or 50 mg	Lopressor HCT
Nadolol 40 or 80 mg/bendroflumethiazide, 5 mg	Corzide
Propranolol hydrochloride 40 or 80 mg/hydrochlorothiazide, 25 mg	Inderide
Propranolol hydrochloride (extended release) 80, 120 or 160 mg/hydrochlorothiazide, 50 mg	Inderide LA
Timolol maleate 10 mg/hydrochlorothiazide, 25 mg	Timolide
ACE inhibitors and diuretics	
Benazepril hydrochloride 5, 10 or 20 mg/hydrochlorothiazide, 6.25, 12.5 or 25 mg	Lotensin HCT
Captopril 25 or 50 mg/hydrochlorothiazide, 15 or 25 mg	Capozide*
Enalaprilmaleate 5 or 10 mg/hydrochlorothiazide, 12.5 or 25 mg	Vaseretic
Lisinopril 10 or 20 mg/hydrochlorothiazide, 12.5 or 25 mg	Prinzide, Zestoretic

Table 6.4 (cont'd)

Angiotensin II receptor antagonists and diuretics	
Losartan potassium 50 mg/hydrochlorothiazide, 12.5 mg	Hyzaar
Valsartan 80 or 160 mg/hydrochlorothiazide, 12.5 mg	Diovan HCT
Calcium antagonists and ACE inhibitors	
Amlodipine besylate 2.5 or 5 mg/benazepril hydrochloride, 10 or 20 mg	Lotrel
Diltiazem hydrochloride 180 mg/enalapril maleate, 5 mg	Teczem
Verapamil hydrochloride (extended release) 180 or 240 mg/trandolapril, 1, 2 or 4 mg	Tarka
Felodipine 5 mg/enalapril maleate, 5 mg	Lexxel
Other combinations	
Triamterene 37.5, 50, or 75 mg/hydrochlorothiazide, 25 or 50 mg	Dyazide, Maxide
Spironolactone 25 or 50 mg/hydrochlorothiazide, 25 or 50 mg	Aldactazide
Amiloride hydrochloride 5 mg/hydrochlorothiazide, 50 mg	Moduretic
Guanethidine monosulfate 10 mg/hydrochlorothiazide, 25 mg	Esimil
Hydralazine hydrochloride 25, 50 or 100 mg/hydrochlorothiazide, 25 or 50 mg	Apresazide
Methyldopa 250 or 500 mg/hydrochlorothiazide, 15, 25 30 or 50 mg	Aldoril
Reserpine 0.125 mg/hydrochlorothiazide, 25 or 50 mg	Hydropres

For example, ACE inhibitors markedly reduce pedal edema associated with dihydropyridine calcium antagonists. Additionally, ACE inhibitors mitigate the adverse lipid and metabolic effects seen with diuretics.

This information, coupled with the fact that in all trials to date combinations of antihypertensive medications have reduced both renal disease progression and cardiovascular events, make the use of combinations of antihypertensive therapy meaningful (10,13,33-35). Differences in cardiovascular outcomes and renal disease progression between monotherapy and combination therapies are summarized in Table 6.5. Thus, the physician may now select agents with complementary modes of action that minimize side effects and maximize compliance in order to achieve better rates of blood pressure control.

Table 6.4 (cont'd)

Other combinations	
Reserpine 0.10 mg/hydralazine hydrochloride, 25 mg/ hydrochlorothiazide, 15 mg	Ser-Ap-Es
Clonidine hydrochloride 0.1, 0.2, or 0.3 mg/chlorthalidone, 15 mg	Combipres
Methyldopa 250 mg/chlorothiazide, 150 or 250 mg	Aldochlor
Reserpine 0.125 or 0.25 mg/chlorthalidone, 25 or 50 mg	Demi-Regroton
Reserpine 0.125 or 0.25 mg/chlorothiazide, 250 or 500 mg	Diupres
Prazosin hydrochloride 1, 2 or 5 mg/polythiazide, 0.5 mg	Minizide

A suggested approach to achieve blood pressure goals is to remember the importance for human as well as physiological factors. From the patients' perspective, there are many factors that can improve adherence with medication regimens. These are reviewed elsewhere but

Table 6.5

The impact of single agent and combination blood pressure lowering strategies on renal and CV outcomes

	CV events	*Renal disease progression*
Single agent		
ACE Inhibitors	Reduced	Markedly slow or stopped
Non-DHPCCBs (verapamil-diltiazem)	Reduced	Markedly slow
DHPCCBs (amlodipine-like)	No reduction ■ Heart failure ■ Type 2 diabetes Reduction ■ ISH*	Slightly slowed – BP reduction effect
β Blockers	Reduced	Slowed
Thiazide diuretics	Reduced	Slowed in diabetic nephropathy
ARBs	Reduced ■ Heart failure	??? (trial results pending)
Combination Therapy		
ACE Inhibitors/ CCBs	Reduced — with and without heart failure or diabetes	Markedly slowed
ACE Inhibitors/ β Blockers	Reduced ■ Heart failure	???
ACE Inhibitors/ diuretics	Reduced	Markedly slowed
β Blockers/ diuretics	Reduced	Slowed

are summarized in Table 6.6. These factors serve to establish a contract with the patient that has been shown to improve medication adherence (2).

Other physiological factors that affect blood pressure such as heart rate also need to be considered. Evidence suggests that resting heart rates of greater than or equal to 84 beats per minute are an independent risk factor for cardiovascular events (36). Thus, in the paradigm to achieve blood pressure goal, agents such as α, β blockers and β blockers have a clear role, Figure 6.4. Combinations of CCBs, in low doses from

Table 6.6

An approach to achieve and maintain blood pressure goals
(1) If BP greater than 15/10 mm Hg ABOVE goal off medications, start with combination therapy, see figure 6.4.
(2) Explain to the patient ALL common side effects and why you selected the particular medication to achieve BP goal, i.e., "it will reduce your risk of stroke, heart attack or kidney failure," and similar explanations.
(3) Explain what the goal BP is and write it down. On a 3x5 card, the LDL cholesterol and HbA1c goals should also be listed. Tell patient that the two of you are responsible to help achieve the BP goals.
Patient responsibilities:
■ report side effects and tolerability issues as well as deviation from regimen
■ measure BP at set time of day, early morning preferable since highest period of cardiovascular risk
■ bring ALL blood pressure readings in at every visit
Physician responsibilities:
■ ask about side effects of medications
■ explore with the patient reasons for lack of adherence, including dietary issues such as high sodium intake, non BP meds (NSAIDs, etc.)
■ identify the BP regimen with the fewest number of pills that will achieve BP goal. In many cases, two different fixed-dose combinations can provide four different medications in two pills

two different subclasses, i.e., diltiazem with nifedipine has been shown to provide synergistic effects on blood pressure reduction (37). Thus, in refractory or difficult to control cases, such combinations should be considered, as exemplified in Table 4.

It should also be noted that ARBs play a role in slowing renal disease progression. However, this data is largely from studies in a heart failure population (38). Renal trial data are not yet available as of this writing. However, ARBs do have a role as agents that lower blood pressure and with their desirable side-effect profile, particularly less hyperkalemia and cough, may be preferred in the future to ACE inhibitors if the trial data support a renoprotective role (39).

Other agents such as alpha blockers have no primary role in blood pressure reduction since they do not reduce mortality (40). Moreover, they have not been shown to reduce albuminuria in people with established nephropathy (41). Thus, this class of agents should be used only as an adjunct to help achieve blood pressure goals.

Concomitant Medications That Attenuate Blood Pressure Lowering

Failure to adequately reduce blood pressure may be a result of multiple factors including secondary causes of hypertension and noncompliance. However, a very common cause of uncontrolled blood pressure is related to the effects of concomitant over-the-counter medications. The two most prevalent types are non-steroidal anti-inflammatory agents, such as ibuprofen, and sympathomimetics, such as pseudoephedrine, in cold preparations. Additionally, oral contraceptive and steroid medications will blunt the antihypertensive effect of most agents. It is of note that in prospective studies, only calcium antagonists and, to a lesser degree, diuretics, maintain their antihypertensive effects in the presence of all these concomitant medications.

Summary

The goal blood pressure reduction for the general population is <140/90 mm Hg and for those with renal disease or diabetes it is <130/80 mm Hg. The approach to achieve this goal is summarized in Figure 6.4. If baseline blood pressure on the initial visit is >15/10 mm Hg above the desired goal, combination therapy will be needed in over 80% of the cases to achieve this goal (42). This observation has been incorporated into the paradigm in Figure 6.4 for initiating therapy.

References:

1. Joint National Committee on Detection, Evaluation, and Treatment of High Blood Pressure. The sixth report of the Joint National Committee on Detection, Evaluation, and Treatment of High Blood Pressure (JNC VI). Arch Intern Med 1997;154: 2413-2446.
2. The National Kidney Foundation Hypertension and Diabetes Executive Committees Working Group. Treatment of Hypertension in Adults with Diabetes to Preserve Renal Function: A consensus approach endorsed by the Scientific Advisory Board of the National Kidney Foundation Am J Kidney Dis, In Press.

3. Feldman RD. The 1999 Canadian recommendations for the management of hypertension. On behalf of the Task Force for the Development of the 1999 Canadian Recommendations for the Management of Hypertension. Can J Cardiol. 1999;15 Suppl G:57G-64G.
4. US Renal Data System: USRDS 1999 Annual Data Report. National Institutes of Health, National Institute of Diabetes & Digestive Kidney Diseases. Bethesda, MD, April 1999.
5. Tarif N and Bakris GL. Pharmacologic treatment of essential hypertension. IN: Johnson R and Freehally J (eds.) Principles of Nephrology Mosby & Co. London, 2000 pp. 40.1-12.
6. Nelson RG, Knowler WC, Pettit DJ, Bennett PH. Kidney disease in diabetes. IN: Diabetes in America, National Institutes of Health Publication No. 95-1468 (2nd edition): 349-400, 1995.
7. Rachmani R, Ravid M. Risk factors for nephropathy in type 2 diabetes mellitus. Compr Ther 1999;25(6-7):366-369.
8. Bakris GL, Walsh MF, Sowers JR. Endothelium/mesangium interactions. Role of insulin-like growth factors . IN: Endocrinology of the Vasculature (Sowers JR, ed). Humana Press Inc. New Jersey, 1996, pp.341-356.
9. Christensen PK, Hansen HP, Parving HH. Impaired autoregulation of GFR in hypertensive non-insulin dependent diabetic patients. Kidney Int 1997;52(5):1369-1374.
10. Peterson JC, Adler S, Burkart JM, Greene T, Hebert LA, Hunsicker LG, King AJ, Massry SG, Seifter JL. Blood pressure control, proteinuria, and the progression of renal disease. The Modification of Diet in Renal Disease Study. Ann Intern Med 1995;123:754-762.
11. Wright JT Jr, Kusek JW, Toto RD, Lee JY, Agodoa LY, Kirk KA, Randall OS, Glassock R. Design and baseline characteristics of participants in the African American Study of Kidney Disease and Hypertension (AASK) Pilot Study. Control Clin Trials 1996;17(4 Suppl):3S-16S.
12. Klag MJ, Whelton PK, Randall BL, Neaton JD, Brancati FL, Ford CE, Shulman NB, Stamler J. Blood pressure and end-stage renal disease in men. N Engl J Med 1996;334:13-18.

13. Effects of intensive blood pressure lowering and low-dose aspirin in patients with hypertension: principal results of the Hypertension Optimal Treatment (HOT) randomized trial. The HOT Study Group. Lancet 1998;351:1755-1762.
14. Estacio RO, Barrett JW, Hiatt WR, Biggerstaff SL, Gifford N, Schrier RW. The effect of nisoldipine as compared with enalapril on cardiovascular outcomes in patients with non-insulin-dependent diabetes and hypertension. N Engl J Med 1998;338:645-652.
15. Tight blood pressure control and risk of macrovascular and microvascular complications in type 2 diabetes: UKPDS 38. UK Prospective Diabetes Study Group. BMJ 1998;317:703-713.
16. Haffner SM, Lehto S, Ronnernaa T, Pyorala K, Laakso M. Mortality from coronary heart disease in subjects with type 2 diabetes and in non-diabetic subjects with and without prior myocardial infarction. N Engl J Med 1998;339:229-234.
17. Borch-Johnsen K, Feldt-Rasmussen B, Strandgaard S, Schroll M, Jensen JS. Urinary albumin excretion. An independent predictor of ischemic heart disease. Arterioscler Thromb Vasc Biol 1999;19:1992-1997.
18. Tuttle KR, Puhlman ME, Cooney SK, Short R. Urinary albumin and insulin as predictors of coronary artery disease: an angiographic study. Am J Kidney Dis 1999;34:918-925.
19. Ravid M, Lang R, Rachmani R, Lishner M. Long-term renoprotective effect of angiotensin-converting enzyme inhibition in non-insulin-dependent diabetes mellitus. A 7-year follow-up study. Arch Intern Med 1996;156:286-289.
20. Keane WF, Eknoyan G. Proteinuria, Albuminuria, Risk Assessment, Detection, Elimination (PARADE): a position paper of the National Kidney Foundation. Am J Kidney Dis 1999; 33:1004-1010.
21. Heart Outcomes Prevention Evaluation (HOPE) Study Investigators. Effects of ramipril on cardiovascular and microvascular outcomes in people with diabetes mellitus: results of the HOPE study and MICRO-HOPE substudy Lancet 2000;355;253-259.
22. Ruggenenti P, Perna A, Benini R, Remuzzi G. Effects of dihydropyridine calcium channel blockers, angiotensin-converting enzyme inhibition, and blood pressure control on chronic, nondiabetic nephropathies. J Am Soc Nephrol 1998;9:2096-2101.

23. Bakris GL, Copley JB, Vicknair N, Sadler R, Leurgans S. Calcium channel blockers versus other antihypertensive therapies on progression of non-insulin-dependent diabetes mellitus associated nephropathy. Kidney Int 1996; 56:1641-1650.

24. Wilmer WA, Hebert LA, Lewis EJ, Rohde RD, Whittier F, Cattran D, Levy AS, Lewis JB, Spitalewitz S, Blumenthal S, Bain RP. Remission of nephrotic syndrome in type 1 diabetes: long term follow-up of patients in the Captopril Study. Am J Kidney Dis 1999;34:308-314.

25. Bakris GL, Mangrum A, Copley JB, Vicknair N, Sadler R. Effect of calcium channel or beta-blockade on the progression of diabetic nephropathy in African Americans. Hypertension 1997;29:744-750.

26. Bakris GL, Weir MR, DeQuattro V, McMahon FG. Effects of an ACE inhibitor/calcium antagonist combination on proteinuria in diabetic nephropathy. Kidney Int 1998;54:1283-1289.

27. Azizi M, Guyene TT, Chatellier G, Wargon M, Menard J. Additive effects of losartan and enalapril on blood pressure and plasma active renin. Hypertension 1997;29:634-640.

28. Tarif N and Bakris GL. Preservation of renal function: the spectrum of effects by calcium channel blockers. Nephrol Dial Transpl 1997;12:2244-2250.

29. Stehouwer CDA, Lambert J, Donker AJM, Van Hinsbergh VWM. Endothelial dysfunction and pathogenesis of diabetic angiopathy. Cardiov Res 1997;34: 55-68.

30. Bakris GL, Weir MR. ACE inhibitor-associated elevations in serum creatinine: Is this a cause for concern? Arch Intern Med 2000;160:685-693.

31. Epstein M and Bakris GL. Newer approaches to antihypertensive therapy: use of fixed dose combination therapy Arch Intern Med 1996;156:1969-1978.

32. Sheinfeld GR, Bakris GL. Benefits of combination angiotensin-converting enzyme inhibitor and calcium antagonist therapy for diabetic patients. Am J Hypertens 1999;12:80S-85S.

33. Jamerson K, Ojo A, Fierro G, HallD, Lawton W, Rahman N, Ram V, Randall O, Shultz P, Steigerwalt S for the HOT Renal Substudy group. Aggressive blood pressure control may eliminate racial disparity in hypertensive renal disease. Am J Hypertens 1999;12:3A.

34. Tuomilehto J, Rastenyte D, Birkenhager WH, Thijs L, Antikainen R, Bulpitt Cj, Fletcher AE, Forette F, Goldhaber A, Palatini P, Sarti C, Fagard R. Effects of calcium-channel blockade in older patients with diabetes and systolic hypertension. Systolic Hypertension in Europe Trial Investigators. N Engl J Med 1999;340(9):677-684.

35. Curb JD, Pressel SL, Cutler JA, Savage PJ, Applegate WB, Black H, Camel G, Davis BR, Frost PH, Gonzalez N, Guthrie G, Oberman A, Rutan GH, Stamler J. Effect of diuretic-based anti-hypertensive treatment on cardiovascular disease risk in older diabetic patients with isolated systolic hypertension. Systolic Hypertension in the Elderly Program Cooperative Research Group. JAMA 1996;276(23):1886-1892.

36. Gillman MW, Kannel WB, Belanger A, DAgostino RB. Influence of heart rate on mortality among persons with hypertension: the Framingham Study. Am Heart J 1993;125:1148-1154.

37. Saseen JJ, Carter BL, Brown TE, Elliott WJ, Black HR. Comparison of nifedipine alone and with diltiazem or verapamil in hypertension. Hypertension 1996;28:109-114.

38. Pitt B, Segal R, Martinez FA, Meurers G, Cowley AJ, Thomas I, Deedwania PC, Ney DE, Snavely DB, Chang PI. Randomized trial of losartan versus captopril in patients over 65 with heart failure (Evaluation of Losartan in the Elderly Study, ELITE): Lancet 1997; 349:747-752.

39. Bakris GL, Siomos M, Richardson D, Janssen I, Bolton WK, Hebert L, Agarwal R, and Catanzaro D for the VAL-K study group. Comparative Effects of an ACE Inhibitor and an Angiotensin Receptor Blocker on Potassium Homeostasis in High Risk Patients Kidney Int, in press.

40. Messerli FH. Implications of discontinuation of doxazosin arm of ALLHAT. Antihypertensive and Lipid-Lowering Treatment to Prevent Heart Attack Trial. Lancet 2000;355(9207):863-864.

41. Rachmani R, Levi Z, Slavachovsky I, Half Onn E, Ravid M. Effect of an alpha-adrenergic blocker, and ACE inhibitor and hydrochlorothiazide on blood pressure and on renal function in type 2 diabetic patients with hypertension and albuminuria. A randomized cross-over study. Nephron 1998;80:175-182.

42. Hilleman DE. Cost-effectiveness of combination therapy. Amer J Managed Care 1999;5:449S-455S.

Management of Heart Failure in the Patient with Diabetes Mellitus

Thomas D. Giles, MD

Heart failure occurs commonly among patients with diabetes for several reasons: diabetes is a risk factor for the development of coronary atherosclerosis and its complications, e.g., myocardial infarction; diabetes is frequently accompanied by hypertension, a factor in the pathogenesis of approximately 70% of heart failure in general; and, the presence of diabetic cardiomyopathy, a disease of heart muscle that is secondary to diabetes, not dependent on the presence of coronary atherosclerosis, and cardioneuropathy. Thus, diabetes is a major risk factor and can contribute in several ways to the development of heart failure. Diabetic cardiomyopathy produces diastolic dysfunction early in the course of the disease (1). Later, symptoms of heart failure may primarily reflect diastolic and systolic ventricular dysfunction. This discussion will be limited to left ventricular systolic dysfunction. General guidelines for the management of left ventricular systolic heart failure have been published (2,3).

Evaluation of the Patient with Diabetes and Heart Failure

As with all patients, the management of heart failure in patients with diabetes depends on an accurate diagnosis and complete medical inventory and assessment of all co-morbidity. Sometimes, the diagnosis of diabetes may be made only after the patient presents with heart failure. The clinician must always be mindful that the presence of diabetes does not protect the patient from other causes of heart failure, e.g., valvular heart disease.

Renal disease is common among patients with diabetes and may render management of heart failure more difficult. Patients with reduced renal function may not respond well to thiazide-type diuretics and larger than usual doses of loop diuretics may be required. Patients with heart failure in general and, diabetes in particular, frequently have abnormal potassium and magnesium balance. Potassium may be low or high, depending on the state of the kidneys. Certain classes of drugs, e.g. potassium sparing diuretics, angiotensin I-converting enzyme/kininase II (ACE/KII) inhibitors, that influence potassium and magnesium balance, merit particularly careful use.

General Management

Most patients with diabetes and heart failure will have type 2 diabetes and obesity. Obesity contributes both to the presence of diabetes and heart failure. Therefore, it is important to have patients with diabetes and heart failure lose weight. Appropriate dietary restrictions and physical exercise are important considerations in designing the treatment of the diabetic patient with heart failure. Table 7.1 outlines general considerations for the management of the patient with diabetes and heart failure.

Table 7.1

General measures for the management of heart failure in diabetes
Measures to decrease the risk of a new cardiac injury (1) cessation of smoking (2) weight reduction in obese patients (3) control of hypertension, hyperlipidemia and diabetes mellitus (4) discontinuation of alcohol use ***Measures to maintain fluid balance*** Patients should restrict their daily intake of salt to a moderate degree (3 grams daily) and should weigh themselves daily to detect the early occurrence of fluid retention. ***Measures to improve physical conditioning*** Patients with heart failure should not be instructed to limit their physical activity; they should be encouraged to engage in moderate degrees of exercise to prevent or reverse physical deconditioning. ***Measures recommended in selected patients*** (1) control of ventricular response in patients with atrial fibrillation or other supraventricular tachycardias (2) anticoagulation in patients with atrial fibrillation or a previous embolic event (and possibly other high-risk patients) (3) coronary revascularization in patients with angina (and possibly, in some patients with ischemic but viable myocardium) ***Pharmacological measures to be avoided*** (1) use of antiarrhythmic agents to suppress asymptomatic ventricular arrhythmias (2) use of most calcium antagonists (3) use of nonsteroidal anti-inflammatory agents ***Other recommended measures*** (1) influenza and pneumococcal immunization (2) close outpatient surveillance to detect early evidence of clinical deterioration

Pharmacological Management of Heart Failure in Diabetes

The principles of pharmacological management of heart failure in diabetes are similar to other patients with heart failure. However, certain aspects of treatment need emphasis and clarification:

- Other specific etiological factors should be sought, e.g. ischemic heart disease (see Chapter III). Hypertension in diabetes is often difficult to control; however, control is necessary to effectively reduce the hemodynamic burden on the heart.
- The strategy to control blood glucose should emphasize weight loss for the obese patient (see Chapter II).
- An assessment of renal function is paramount. Patients with diabetes may exhibit nephrotic range proteinuria; a subsequent in reduction in serum albumin confounds clinical assessment of intravascular volume status. Also, marked reduction in glomerular filtration may be present as indicated by elevation in serum creatinine and blood urea nitrogen. Hyperkalemia, associated with type 4 renal tubular acidosis may make use of certain drug classes, e.g. ACE/kininase II inhibitors, difficult. Patients with diabetes and heart failure who have marked renal impairment will usually require referral to a specialty group with management performed by both a cardiologist and a nephrologist.

- The hemodynamic burden of the heart should be reduced. This unloading of the heart may be accomplished by reducing heart rate and blood pressure and reducing the demand for an increased cardiac output and myocardial contractility.
- The process of cardiac remodeling should be thwarted by administration of drugs that target the pathophysiological cascade common to virtually all advanced cardiomyopathies with heart failure.

Currently, four classes of drugs are approved for the treatment of heart failure. This approval is based on clinical trial evidence; all of the clinical trials contained patients with diabetes and thus the evidence may be extended to this group. These classes are: diuretics, angiotensin I-converting enzyme (ACE/kininase II) inhibitors, beta-adrenoceptor antagonists (beta-blockers), and cardiac glycosides (digoxin, digitoxin) (Table 7.2). Despite clinical trial experience, confusion still exists regarding the use of these drugs in patients with diabetes; some of these confusing aspects will be discussed. An algorithm which may be useful is presented in Figure 7.1.

Diuretics

Diuretics are the mainstay of treatment for patients with excess intra- or extravascular volume (peripheral or pulmonary edema). Diuretics are often the first drugs administered to patients with heart failure if an increased volume status is diagnosed, i.e., in the presence of high systemic venous pressures (elevated jugular venous pressure) and pulmonary or systemic edema (4,5). In the patient with diabetes, in particular, caution must be exercised in assessing the intravascular volume status until the serum albumin concentration is measured, i.e., the edema may be due to a reduced serum oncotic pressure, as well as increased capillary permeability associated with diabetes. A skillful assessment of the venous pressure by inspection of the neck veins is invaluable for the clinician in determining intravascular volume status.

For urgent or emergent situations, the loop diuretics are often used first and often given by a parenteral route. In diabetic patients with reduced renal function these drugs may be required in larger than usual doses. The loop diuretics have a short duration of action, i.e., 4 to 6 hours (except for torsemide). For long-term administration, the thiazide diuretics may be preferred, particularly if renal function is not too compromised; also, the thiazide diuretics augment the effects of the loop diuretics since they act proximally and distally to the loop of Henle. For patients with hypertension and diabetes, thiazide diuretics may offer an additional antihypertensive mechanism.

The "potassium-sparing" diuretics act by antagonizing the effects of aldosterone on the kidney. This action is helpful in preventing the depletion of potassium and magnesium, which often accompanies both heart failure and diabetes. The recent Randomized Aldactone Evaluation Study (RALES) trial suggests that spironolactone may be useful as a part of the initial diuretic regimen, since antagonism of aldosterone produces other benefits as well, e.g. alteration of cardiac remodeling in patients with advanced heart failure (6). As indicated above, in the patient with diabetes, caution must be exercised so as not to produce hyperkalemia. In this latter regard, attention must be paid to the administration of potassium supplements or ACE inhibitors.

Diuretics should generally not be used as monotherapy in patients with heart failure. Diuretics activate the renin-angiotensin-aldosterone system and contribute to electrolyte disturbances and arrhythmias. The dose of diuretics should be adjusted as frequently as necessary to maintain optimal volume status. Daily recording of body weight is greatly helpful in achieving this goal.

Table 7.2 **(continued on next page)**

Drugs frequently used for treatment of heart failure

Class	*Generic name*	*Usual dosage*
Diuretics		
Thiazide-like	Chlorothiazide	500-1000 mg PO, IV
	Hydrochlorothiazide	25-100 mg PO
	Indapamide	2.5-5 mg PO
	Metolazone	2.5-20 mg PO
Loop diuretics	Furosemide	10-240 mg PO, IV
	Ethacrynic acid	50-100 mg PO, IV
	Bumetanide	5-10 mg PO, IV
	Torsemide	10-20 mg PO, IV
Potassium-sparing	Amiloride	5-20 mg PO
	Spironolactone	25-400 mg PO
	Triamterene	100-300 mg PO
Carbonic anhydrase inhibitor	Acetazolamide	250-500 mg PO

PO = per os; IV = intravenously; SL = sublingually

Table 7.2 (cont'd)

Drugs frequently used for treatment of heart failure		
Class	***Generic name***	***Usual dosage***
ACE inhibitors	Captopril	6.25-50 mg PO tid
	Enalapril	2.5-20 mg PO bid
	Lisinopril	2.5-20 mg PO qd
	Quinapril	5-20 mg PO bid
	Fosinopril	20-40 mg PO qd
	Ramipril	2.5-20 mg qd
Beta blockers	Carvedilol	3.125 mg bid *
	Bisoprolol	1.25 qd *
	Metoprolol	5 mg bid *
	Metoprolol XL	12.5 mg qd *
Direct-acting vasodilators	Isosorbide dinitrate	2.5-60 mg PO tid-qid
	Hydralazine	10-75 mg PO tid-qid
	Nitroprusside	5-150 μ/min IV
	Nitroglycerin	10-500 μ/min IV 5-60 mg/PO tid-qid 0.3-0.8 mg SL
Cardiac glycoside	Digoxin	0.125-0.375 mg PO qd
Inotropes	Dobutamine	2.5-20.0 μg/kg/min IV
	Dopamine	2-10 μg/kg/min IV
	Amrinone	bolus 0.75-2.0 mg/kg; IV maintenance 5-20 μg/kg/min
	Milrinone	bolus 50 μg/kg maintenence 0.375-0.75 μg/kg/min
Calcium antagonists	Amlodipine	5-10 mg PO qd
	Felodipine	30-120 mg PO qd 180-300 mg CD qd

* Doses obtained from the following studies: CIBIS, MERIT-HF, MDC, and the carvedilol trials.

Figure 7.1

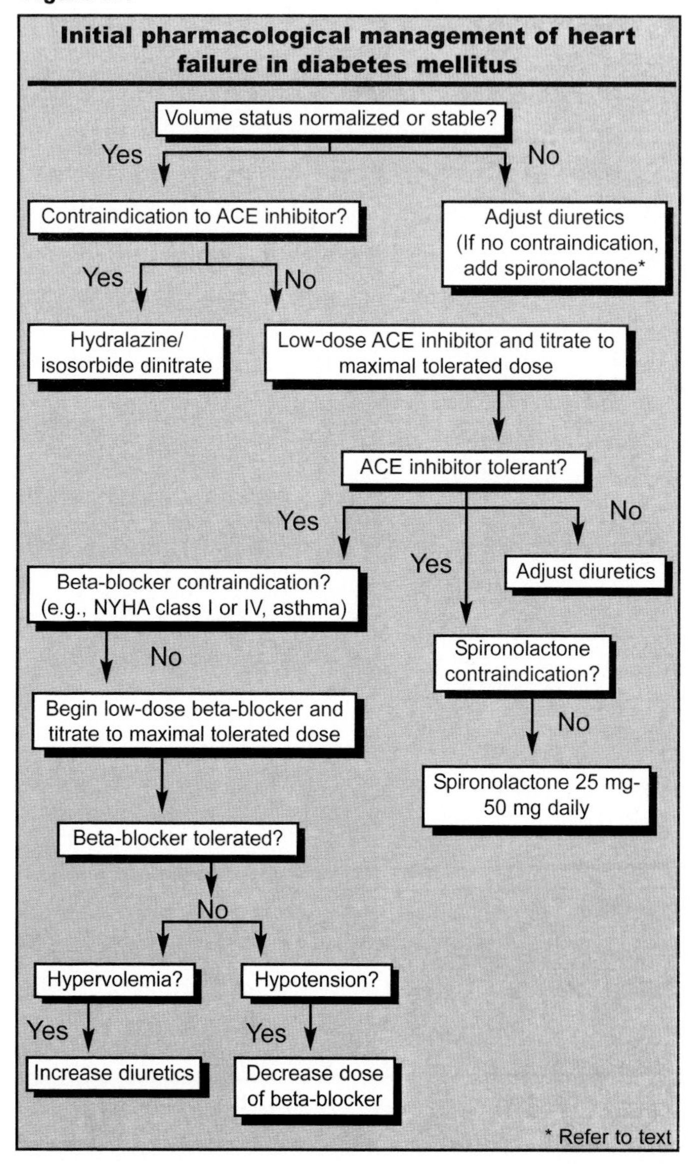

Initial pharmacological management of heart failure in diabetes mellitus
Volume status normalized or stable?
Yes
No
Contraindication to ACE inhibitor?
Adjust diuretics (If no contraindication, add spironolactone*
Yes
No
Hydralazine/ isosorbide dinitrate
Low-dose ACE inhibitor and titrate to maximal tolerated dose
ACE inhibitor tolerant?
Yes
No
Yes
Adjust diuretics
Beta-blocker contraindication? (e.g., NYHA class I or IV, asthma)
No
Spironolactone contraindication?
Begin low-dose beta-blocker and titrate to maximal tolerated dose
No
Spironolactone 25 mg-50 mg daily
Beta-blocker tolerated?
No
Hypervolemia?
Hypotension?
Yes
Yes
Increase diuretics
Decrease dose of beta-blocker
* Refer to text

Angiotensin I–Converting Enzyme (ACE)/ Kininase II Inhibitors

ACE/kininase II inhibitors should be administered to all patients with impaired left ventricular function, regardless of whether or not symptoms are present, unless a contraindication to their use is present, e.g. angioedema. This recommendation is based on a large amount of clinical trial data that has demonstrated both efficacy and safety of these drugs (7,8,9,10,11,12). ACE inhibitors reduce symptoms of heart failure, e.g. dyspnea and fatigue, and prolong life. ACE inhibitors also reduce the progression of heart failure in patients who are asymptomatic.

The ACE inhibitors may be of particular benefit to patients with diabetes and heart failure since upregulation of the enzyme occurs in diabetes. The HOPE trial indicated that a reduction in heart failure occurred in patients receiving an ACE inhibitor (13).

The initial dose of an ACE inhibitor should be low for older patients and those who have low blood pressures or have been aggressively diuresed. For patients with an acute myocardial infarction, particularly diabetic patients, ACE inhibitors should be started as soon as possible unless the patient is hemodynamically unstable or has a contraindication to use (14,15,16,17,18). ACE inhibitor administration may be associated with an increase in serum creatinine, particularly in patients with impaired renal function as may exist with diabetes and hypertension. However, a small increase in serum creatinine should not be a cause of great concern and if necessary, a reduction in diuretics should be the first corrective step. The changes in renal function that occur in patients with heart failure following administration of ACE inhibitors are secondary to the decrease in blood pressure and the selective dilation of the efferent arteriole of the glomerulus and are not due to a "toxic" effect on the kidney. In some patients with diabetes, ACE inhibitors may trigger a response that may be similar to that seen in renal artery stenosis, in a sharp rise in serum creatinine. In particular, concomitant treatment with a non-steroidal anti-inflammatory drug (NSAID) should be avoided.

ACE inhibitors should be titrated to the maximally tolerated dose. The beneficial influence of higher doses of ACE inhibitors in heart failure was shown in the Assessment of Treatment with Lisinopril and Survival (ATLAS) trial (19).

ACE inhibitors are well-tolerated drugs. Cough may be an adverse side effect of these drugs and in some patients may limit the use of these agents. However, cough is also a symptom of heart failure. Therefore, the presence of a cough in a patient with heart failure may not prepresent a side effect of medication, but may indicate a worsening of the clinical condition. The ACE inhibitor cough characteristically originates in the upper airway (often the posterior pharynx) and worsens at night. Patients often use an "open hand over the throat" to indicate the source of the cough.

Beta Blockers

Two of the great pharmacological myths of the past involve the use of beta blockers: beta blockers are contraindicated in heart failure and, beta blockers are contraindicated in patients with diabetes mellitus. There are now more clinical trial data to recommend the use of beta blockers in heart failure than exist for ACE inhibitors (20,21,22,23,24,25,26,27). Beta blockers are indicated for patients with diabetes and heart failure who are class II to III (New York Heart Association) after ACE inhibitors have been titrated to maximum doses. Beta blocker therapy should be considered even for patients who are intolerant to ACE inhibitors. Beta blockers should not be used in patients who are in a volume overload status, or who have severe hemodynamic compromise. In particular, patients with advanced (Class IV, NYHA) disease may not be able to tolerate even small doses of beta blockers. The initial dose of a beta blocker should be small and titration should occur over 8 to 26 weeks, depending on the particular beta blocker chosen. Similar to ACE inhibitors, beta blockers should be administered to patients with acute myocardial infarction as soon as possible. Again, patients with diabetes will benefit the most.

Improvement in cardiac function requires some time, weeks or months, after the initiation of beta blocker therapy. In fact, the initiation of beta blocker therapy in heart failure may be accompanied by a worsening of symptoms, symptomatic hypotension, or severe bradycardia. Volume overload, as evidenced by abnormal jugular venous pressure, or edema, may require augmentation of diuretic therapy. Beta blocker therapy may require a reduction or discontinuance of treatment with amiodarone or digoxin.

Digoxin

Digoxin therapy may be used in patients with heart failure if, after treatment with diuretics, ACE inhibitors, and beta blockers, symptoms of heart failure persist, e.g. dyspnea and fatigue (28). There are no published data specific to the use of digoxin in patients with diabetes and heart failure. Digoxin improves the symptoms of heart failure but does not influence duration of life (29). Digoxin may be indicated early in the therapeutic course for patients with heart failure accompanied by atrial fibrillation.

Hydralazine/Isosorbide-Dinitrate

The combination of hydralazine/isosorbide-dinitrate improves both symptoms and duration of life in patients with heart failure (30). It is not certain if these drugs are more or less effective in patients with diabetes. However, diabetes is viewed as a nitric oxide deficient state and therefore, the addition of a nitrate may be of particular benefit to people with type 2 diabetes. For patients who are intolerant to ACE inhibitors, the combination may offer an alternative treatment. The combination may also be useful for patients with heart failure and who are difficult to treatment hypertension.

Other Drugs

The third-generation dihydropyridine calcium antagonists, e.g. amlodipine and felodipine, may be useful if a need for further vasodilation arises after treatment with the standard drugs used for heart failure. Treatment with calcium channel blockers does not confer a survival benefit (31,32,33).

The use of the angiotensin II (AT_1) receptor antagonists has not been established for improving survival in patients with heart failure (34). However, these drugs have been shown to improve symptoms in patients with heart failure and may offer additional benefit for patients taking ACE inhibitors (35-45) No specific data are available for the use of angiotensin II (AT_1) receptor antagonists in diabetic patients with heart failure.

As mentioned above, the aldosterone antagonist spironolactone may be useful in patients with heart failure, over and above, the benefits derived from its diuretic properties. Aldosterone may contribute to pathological remodeling of the heart and blockade of this effect may be responsible for the mortality benefit seen in the RALES trial.

Summary

The approach to the pharmacological treatment of patients with diabetes and heart failure is similar to that of heart failure alone. Certain aspects of diagnosis and treatment that are peculiar to diabetes require attention, particular the obscure nature of coronary atherosclerosis, presence of renal disease and electrolyte problems and the co-morbidity of hypertension. It should be remembered that the mainstays of treatment of heart failure, i.e., ACE inhibitors and beta blockers, are of particular benefit for the patient with diabetes. Therefore, the patient with diabetes has much to gain from a careful approach to diagnosis and treatment of heart failure.

References:

1. Dhalla NS, Pierce GN, Innes IR, Beamish RE. Pathogenesis of cardiac dysfunction in diabetes mellitus. Can J Cardiol 1:263-281, 1985.
2. Heart Failure: Management of Patients with Left Ventricular Systolic Dysfunction. Clinical Practice Guideline, Quick Reference Guide for Clinicians. U.S. Department of Health and Human Services. Public Health Service Agency for Health Care Policy and Research: AHCPR Publication No. 94-0613, 1994.
3. Packer M, Cohn JH, eds. Consensus Recommendations for the management of chronic heart failure: Am J Cardiol, 1999; 83:1A.
4. Brater DC Diuretic therapy: N Engl J Med; 1998, 339:387.
5. Richardson A. Bayliss J. Scriven A.J., et al. Double-blind comparison of captopril alone against furosemide plus amiloride in mild heart failure: Lancet, 1987, 2:709.
6. Pitt B. Zannand, F. Remme WJ et al. The effect of spironolactone on morbidity and mortality in patients with severe heart failure: N Engl J Med: 1999, 341:709.
7. SOLVD Investigators: Effect of enalapril on survival in patients with reduced left ventricular ejection fractions and congestive heart failure; N Engl J Med: 1991, 325:293.

8. Captopril Multicenter Research Group. A placebo-controlled trial of captopril in refractory chronic congestive heart failure; J Am Coll Cardiol: 1983, 2:755.
9. The Captopril-Digoxin Multicenter Research Group. Comparative effects of therapy with captopril and digoxin in patients with mild to moderate heart failure; JAMA: 1988, 259:539.
10. Sharpe DN, Murphy J. Coson R, et al. Enalapril in patients with chronic heart failure: a placebo-controlled, randomized, double-blind study; Circulation: 1984, 70:271.
11. The CONSENSUS Trial Study Group. Effects of enalapril on mortality in severe congestive heart failure. Results of the Cooperative North Scandinavian Enalapril Survival Study (CONSENSUS); N Engl J Med: 1987, 316:1429.
12. Giles TD, Katz R. Sullivan JM, et al, for the Multicenter Lisinopril-Captopril Congestive Heart Failure Study Group. Short and long acting angiotensin-converting enzyme inhibitors: A randomized trial of lisinopril versus captopril in the treatment of congestive heart failure; J Am Coll Cardiol: 1989, 13:1240.
13. Heart Outcomes Prevention Evaluation (HOPE) Study Investigators. Effects of captopril in cardiovascular and microvascular outcomes in people with diabetes mellitus benefits the HOPE Study and MICRO-HOPE Substudy; Lancet: 2000, 355:253-9.
14. ISIS Collaborative Group. ISIS-4: A randomised factorial trial assessing early oral captopril, oral mononitrate, and intravenous magnesium sulphate in 58,050 patients with suspected acute myocardial infarction; Lancet: 1995, 345:669.
15. Pfeffer MA, Braunwald E. Moye LA, et al. Effect of captopril on mortality and morbidity in patients with left ventricular dysfunction after myocardial infarction. Results of the Survival and Ventricular Enlargement trial; N Engl J Med: 1992, 327:669.
16. Gruppo Italiano per lo Studio della Sopravvivenza nell'Infarto Miocardico GISSI-3: Effects of lisinopril and transdermal glyceryl trinitrate singly and together on a 6-week mortality and ventricular function after acute myocardial infarction; Lancet: 1994, 343:1115.

17. Chinese Cardiac Study Collaborative Group. Oral captopril versus placebo among 13,634 patients with suspected acute myocardial infarction. Interim report from the Chinese Cardiac Study (CCS-1); Lancet: 1995, 345:686.
18. ACE Inhibitor Myocardial Infarction Collaborative Group. Indications for ACE inhibitors in the early treatment of acute myocardial infarction. Systematic over view of individual data from 100,000 patients in randomized trials: Circulation: 1998, 97:2202.
19. Cleland JFG, Armstrong P. Horowitz JD, et al. on behalf of the ATLAS Investigators. Baseline clinical characteristics of patients recruited into the Assessment of Treatment with Lisinopril and Survival Study (ATLAS) (unpublished data).
20. Fisher ML Gottlieb SS; Plotnick GD, et al. Beneficial effects of metoprolol in heart failure associated with coronary artery disease: A randomized trial; J Am Coll Cardiol: 1994, 23:943.
21. Merit-HF Study Group. Effect of metoprolol CR/XL in chronic heart failure: Metoprolol CR/XL. Randomized Intervention Trial in Congestive Heart Failure (MERIT-HF); Lancet: 1999, 353:2001.
22. Olsen SL, Gilbert EM, Renlund DG, et al. Carvedilol improves left ventricular function symptoms in chronic heart failure: A double-blind randomized study; J Am Coll Cardiol: 1995, 25:1225.
23. Krum H. Sackner-Bernstein JD, Goldsmith RL, et al. Double-blind, placebo-controlled study of the long term efficacy of carvedilol in patients with severe chronic heart failure; Circulation: 1995, 92:1499.
24. Waagstein F, Bristow MR, Swedberg K, et al, for the Metoprolol in Dilated Cardiomyopathy (MDC) Trial Study Group. Beneficial effects of metoprolol in idiopathic dilated cardiomyopathy; Lancet: 1993, 342:1441.
25. Colucci WS, Packer M, Bristow MR et al, for the US Carvedilol Heart Failure Study Group. Carvedilol inhibits clinical progression in patients with mild symptoms of heart failure; Circulation: 1996, 94:2800.

26. CIBIS II Investigators and Committees. The Cardiac Insufficiency Bisoprolol Study (CIBIS-II): A randomised trial; Lancet: 1999, 353:9.

27. Packer M, Bristow MR, Cohn JN, et al, for the US Carvedilol Heart Failure Study Group. The effect of carvedilol on morbidity and mortality in patients with chronic heart failure; N Engl J Med: 1996, 334:1349.

28. Hauptman, PJ, Kelly RA. Digitalis; Circulation: 1999, 99:1265.

29. The Digitalis Investigation Group. The effect of digoxin on mortality and morbidity in patients with heart failure; N Engl J Med: 1997, 336:525.

30. Cohn JN, Archibald DG, Ziesche S, et al. Effect of vasodilator therapy on mortality of a Veterans Administration Cooperative Study; N Engl J Med: 1986, 14:1547.

31. Packer M, O'Connor CM, Ghali JK, et al. Effect of amlodipine on morbidity and mortality in severe chronic heart failure; N Engl J Med: 1996, 335:1107.

32. Cohn JN, Ziesche S, Smith R, et al. Effect of the calcium antagonist felodipine as supplementary vasodilator therapy in patients with chronic heart failure treated with enalapril. V-HeFT III; Circulation: 1997, 96:856.

33. Packer M, O'Conner CM, Ghali JK, Pressler ML, Carson PE, Belkin RN, Miller AB, Neuberg GW, Frid D, Wertheimer JH, Cropp AB, DeMets DL. Effect of amlodipine on morbidity and mortality in severe chronic heart failure. Prospective Randomized Amlodipine Survival Evaluation Study Group. N Engl J Med. 1996 Oct 10;335(15):1107-14.

34. Sander GE, McKinnie JJ, Greenberg SS, Giles TD. Angiotensin-converting enzyme inhibitors and angiotensin II receptor antagonists in the treatment of heart failure caused by left ventricular systolic dysfunction. Prog Cardiovasc Dis. 1999 Jan-Feb;41(4):265-300.

35. Gottlieb SS, Dickstein DK, Fleck E, et al. Hemodynamic and neurohormonal effects of the angiotensin II antagonist losartan patients with congestive heart failure; Circulation: 1993, 88:1602.

36. Crozier I, Ikram H, Awan N, et al. Losartan in heart failure. Hemodynamic effects and tolerability; Circulation: 1995, 91:691.

37. Lang RM, Elkayam U, Yellen LG, et al, on behalf of the Losartan Pilot Exercise Study Investigators. Comparative effects of losartan and enalapril on exercise capacity and clinical status in patients with heart failure; J Am Coll Cardiol: 1997, 30:983.

38. Pitt B, Segal R, Martinez FA et al. Randomized trial of losartan versus captopril in patients over 65 with heart failure (Evaluation of Losartan in The Elderly study, ELITE); Lancet: 1997, 349:747.

39. Vijay N, Alhaddad IA, Marty Denny D, et al. Irbesartan compared with lisinopril in patients with mild to moderate heart failure; J Am Coll Cardiol: 1998, 31(suppl A):68A.

40. Hamroff G, Glaufarb I, Mancini D, et al. Angiotensin II-receptor blockade further reduces afterload safely in patients maximally treated with angiotensin-converting enzyme inhibitors for heart failure; Journal of Cardiovascular Pharmacology: 1997, 30:458.

41. Baruch L, Anand IS, Judd DL, et al, for Valsartan Study Group. Hemodynamic response to AT(1) receptor blockade with valsartan in ACE inhibitor-treated patients with heart failure; Circulation: 1996, 94(suppl):I-428.

42. Yasuf S, Maggioni AP, Held P. et al. Effects of candesartan, enalapril or their combination on exercise capacity, ventricular function, clinical deterioration and quality of life in heart failure; Randomized Evaluation of Strategies for Left Ventricular Dysfunction (RESOLVD); Circulation: 1998, 96(suppl):I-452.

43. Tocchi M. Rosanio S, Anzuini A, et al. Angiotensin II receptor blockage combined to ACE inhibition improves left ventricular dilation and exercise ejection fraction in congestive heart failure; J Am Coll Cardiol; 1998: 31(suppl A):188A.

44. Tonkon M, Awan N, Niazi I, et al. Irbesartan combined with conventional therapy, including angiotensin converting enzyme inhibitors, in heart failure; J Am Coll Cardiol: 1998, 31 (suppl A):188A.

45. Hamroff G, Blaufarb I, Mancini D, et al. Clinical benefits of long-term angiotensin II receptor blockade in patients with severe symptoms of congestive heart failure despite full angiotensin converting enzyme inhibition; J Am Coll Cardiol: 1998, 31(suppl A):188A.

Special Considerations in Glucose-Lowering Strategies in Patients with Cardiovascular Diseases

Peter A. Brady, MD

Introduction

Non-insulin dependent (type 2) diabetes mellitus is a major independent risk factor for the development of coronary artery disease with a more than three-fold increase in the incidence of acute coronary syndromes and congestive heart failure, even after adjustment for multiple risk factors (1,2). It has been estimated that up to one-third of patients with diabetes are affected by major cardiovascular events on long-term follow-up (3,4). Diabetics also have an increased incidence of late complications and decreased survival following acute myocardial infarction and coronary interventions such as coronary angioplasty, despite similar rates of patency of the "culprit" vessel or initial angiographic results indistinguishable from patients without diabetes (5,6,7).

While many factors are believed to impact morbidity and mortality among patients with diabetes mellitus (Fig. 8.1), one important contributor may be the use of sulfonylurea drugs in some patients (8). Better understanding of whether use of sulfonylurea drugs is potentially harmful is crucial to the management of patients with diabetes and cardiovascular disease since sulfonylureas are the most commonly used oral hypoglycemic agents in clinical practice (9,10).

The purpose of this chapter is to discuss the background, as well as experimental and clinical evidence, for potentially harmful effects of sulfonylurea drugs, a phenomenon recently termed "the sulfonylurea controversy" (11).

Historical Background

Sulfonylurea drugs were introduced into clinical practice in the early 1960s, and for many years were the sole treatment for patients with non-insulin dependent diabetes mellitus. However, publication of the University Group Diabetes Program (UGDP) trial generated

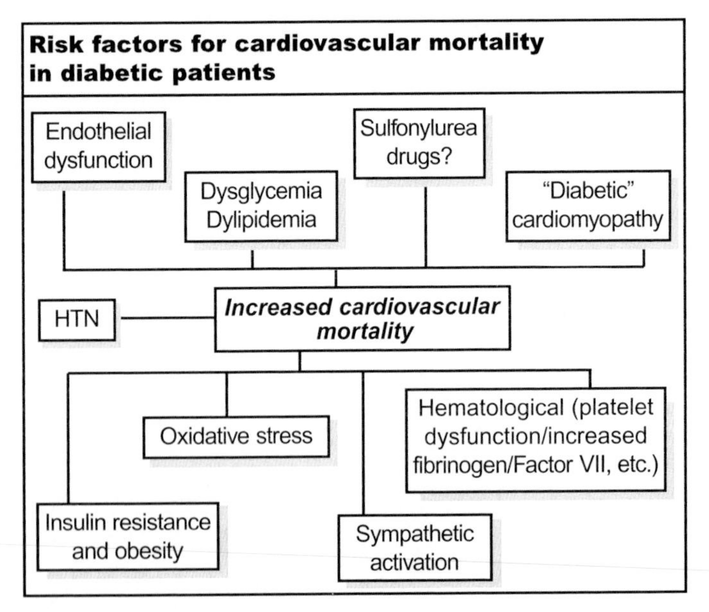

Figure 8.1. Sulfonylurea-drugs are among many factors that may impact cardiovascular outcomes in diabetic patients.

considerable controversy regarding the potential adverse cardiovascular effects of sulfonylurea drugs among patients with diabetes mellitus (12). This trial (one of the first multi-center prospective trials of its kind) reported a substantially increased cardiovascular mortality among patients treated with the sulfonylurea drug, tolbutamide. At that time, however, the mechanism by which sulfonylurea drugs might increase cardiovascular mortality was not apparent. Despite significant criticism of the methodology used in the trial (13), the safety of sulfonylurea drugs in diabetic patients with cardiovascular disease was questioned. Over 30 years later, the controversy and uncertainty regarding safe use of sulfonylurea drugs among patients with diabetes and cardiac disease still remains unresolved (8,11).

A Possible Mechanism of Adverse Cardiovascular Effects of Sulfonylurea-drugs

In the last two decades, considerable progress has been made in the field of cellular electrophysiology and in understanding the function of ion-channels, including cardiac ion-channels (11). One important finding was the discovery of the site of action of sulfonylurea drugs that act on specialized cells in the pancreas known as beta cells (Fig. 8.2). Sulfonylurea drugs exert their hypoglycemic action through inhibition of an ion-channel protein located on the membrane surface of pancreatic beta cells (Fig. 8.2). Inhibition of this channel (ATP sensitive K^+ (KATP) channel), through binding of the sulfonylurea drug to a specific receptor (known as the sulfonylurea receptor (14)) associated with the channel pore complex, leads to depolarization of the beta cell membrane, release of intra-cellular calcium stores and secretion of insulin.

It was known from earlier work that myocardial cells also possess an abundance of sarcolemmal KATP channels that are regulated by intracellular ATP (15). In the presence of high ATP levels (during basal cell metabolism) the KATP channel is kept closed. However, during periods of cellular hypoxia, when the levels of ATP fall, ATP inhibition of the KATP channel

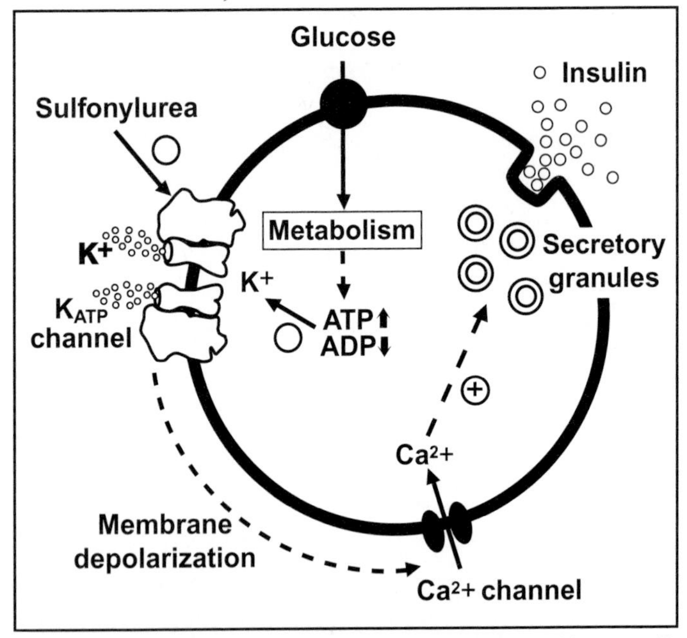

Figure 8.2. Sulfonylurea-drugs act through binding with a specific receptor associated with a metabolic sensitive ion channel (ATP-sensitive potassium channel). Inhibition of this channel leads to depolarization of the cell membrane, release of stored calcium and secretion of insulin.

is lost allowing an outward K^+ current and shortening of the cardiac cell action potential duration. At the cellular level, sulfonylurea drugs also cause accelerated calcium loading within hypoxic cardiac cells which leads rapidly to cell death presumably through inhibition of the cellular protective effects of KATP channels (16). Although the precise significance of these experimental findings are not fully understood, KATP channels do appear to possess significant cardioprotective properties, acting to protect cells from ischemic injury (17). The process by which opening of KATP channels protect the myocardium from ischemic injury is known as ischemic preconditioning (Fig. 8.3) (18). Blockade of KATP channels by sulfonylurea drugs, leading to loss of the cardioprotective response, could be the basis for increased cardiovascular mortality observed in the UGDP study (8, 11).

Do Sulfonylurea Drugs Impair Ischemic Pre-conditioning in Humans?

In one of the first demonstrations of the phenomenon of ischemic pre-conditioning in humans, Murray et al (19) used sequential balloon inflations in a group of patients undergoing coronary angioplasty. Using this model they were able to demonstrate improvement in clinical indicators of ischemia severity with subsequent balloon inflations. It has also been observed that in some patients with myocardial infarction the presence of pre-infarction angina is associated with reduced infarct size, improved ventricular function, and lower in-hospital

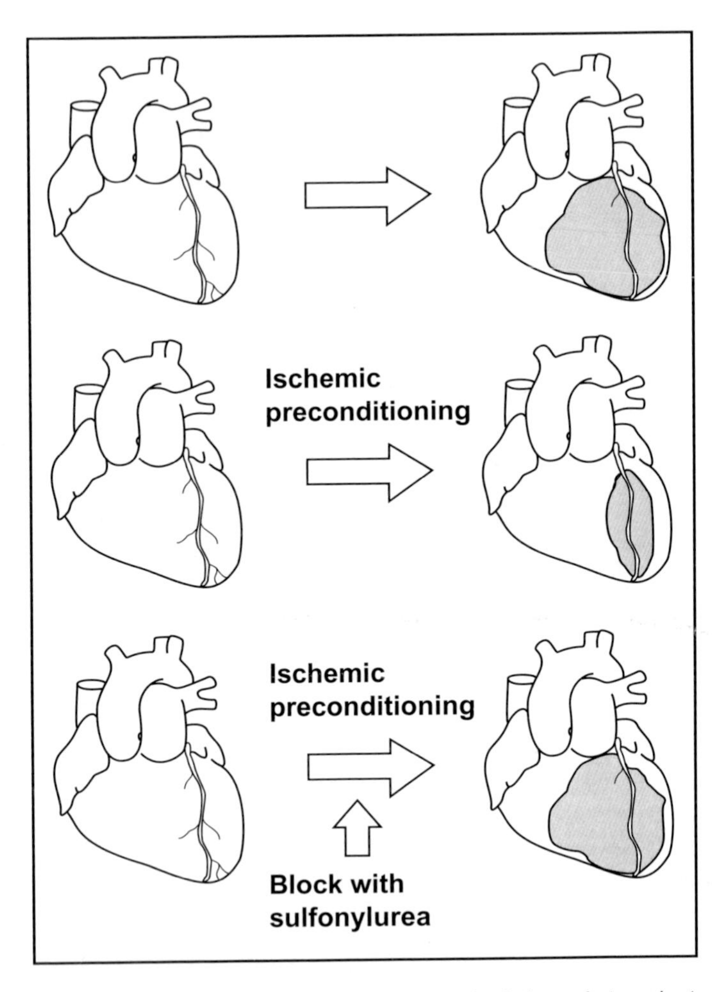

Figure 8.3. Ischemic preconditioning invoked through transient ischemic episodes may protect the myocardium leading to a decrease in the size of myocardial infarction following coronary occlusion. This process of endogenous cardioprotection is inhibited by sulfonylurea-drugs.

mortality compared to patients without pre-infarct angina. In contrast, loss of the pre-conditioning response has consistently been observed in the presence of sulfonylurea drugs (8,11). In a recent retrospective study of patients undergoing direct angioplasty for treatment of acute myocardial infarction, use of sulfonylurea drugs was an independent predictor of mortality with an adverse outcome similar to that associated with a diagnosis of congestive heart failure (20).

The notion that sulfonylurea drugs are harmful to patients with cardiac disease must be balanced, however, against extensive clinical experience with sulfonylureas in diabetic patients which points to the benefit of optimal glucose control. For example, the recently published United Kingdom Prospective Diabetes Study (UKPDS), the largest prospective outcome trial of patients with non-insulin dependent (type 2) diabetes mellitus, demonstrates the benefits of glycemic control (4). Although UKPDS was not designed to directly compare sulfonylurea drug treatment with other therapeutic strategies, no increase in mortality, myocardial infarction, or other cardiovascular event was found among patients treated with sulfonylurea drugs. One explanation for the fewer cardiovascular events observed among patients taking sulfonylurea drugs in the UKPDS trial is that patients were recruited early in the course of their disease (unlike UDGP), prior to the development of significant atherosclerosis. Despite this limitation, follow-up studies of patients following myocardial infarction treated with sulfonylurea drugs have also not demonstrated an increase in mortality, or the extent of myocardial necrosis (21,22).

Overall, the controversy surrounding use of sulfonylurea drugs in patients with diabetes and cardiac disease has made clinical decision-making regarding the best management of such patients (who would otherwise be good candidates for sulfonylurea drugs) difficult. This difficulty has intensified the search for alternative approaches to managing these patients. In this regard is the renewed interest among some investigators in the potential benefit of either continuous glucose infusion, followed by intensive insulin treatment, or glucose insulin and potassium (GIK) infusion in both patients with and without diabetes (23,24,25,26). It remains to be determined, however, whether improved outcomes observed in patients treated with insulin infusion or GIK derives from their metabolic effect, improved glycemic control or from withdrawal of sulfonylurea drugs.

Should Sulfonylurea Drugs be Used in Diabetic Patients with Cardiac Disease?

The major question for cardiologists in treating patients with non-insulin dependent diabetes mellitus is whether sulfonylurea drugs should be discontinued in those patients with significant cardiovascular disease. Unfortunately, at this time no clear guidelines exist to help answer this. In practical terms, sulfonylureas are beneficial in most patients with type 2 diabetes and data related to the adverse cardiovascular effects of sulfonylurea drugs, although compelling, is not proven. On the basis of available data, sulfonylurea drugs do not appear to increase mortality in most patients with diabetes who have stable cardiac disease on long-term follow-up. However, given the experimental and clinical data that sulfonylurea drugs may impair endogenous cardioprotective mechanisms, it would seem prudent to discontinue these agents in high risk patients and control hyperglycemia with insulin, or another agent, until myocardial ischemia has been resolved. Following clinical stabilization, the sulfonylurea could then probably be restarted safely. The role of metabolic approaches to diabetic patients using infusions such as GIK remains to be determined in larger clinical trials.

Conclusions

Experimental evidence and clinical experience suggests that sulfonylurea drugs impair endogenous cardioprotective mechanisms that protect the heart from ischemic insult. However, the consequences of these actions in selected patients are unknown. Although early clinical studies suggested an increased cardiovascular mortality among patients taking sulfonylurea drugs, this finding has not been born out in more recent trials. In light of conflicting data, and lack of clear guidelines on the management of diabetic patients with cardiac disease taking sulfonylurea drugs, the approach to such patients should be individualized. Where possible, alternative strategies for lowering blood glucose should be used especially in those patients with active or significant cardiac ischemia. Use of aggressive metabolic approaches to patients with myocardial ischemia, such as the use of GIK infusion, is promising but requires further study.

References:

1. Uusitupa M, Nikanen LK, Siitonen O, et al. Ten-year cardiovascular mortality in relation to risk factors and abnormalities in lipoprotein composition in type-2 (non-insulin-dependent) diabetic and non-diabetic subjects. Diabetologica 1993;36:1175-84.
2. Stamler J, Vaccaro O, Neaton JD et al. Diabetes, other risk factors, and 12 year cardiovascular mortality for men screened in the Multiple Risk Factor Intervention Trial. Diabetes Care 1993;16:434-444.
3. Laakso M, Lehto S. Epidemiology of macrovascular disease in diabetes. Diabetes Reviews 1997;5:294-315.
4. UKPDS. Intensive blood-glucose control with sulphonylureas or insulin compared with conventional treatment and risk of complications in patients with Type 2 diabetes. Lancet 1998;352:837-853.
5. Granger C, Califf RM, Young S et al. Outcome of patients with diabetes mellitus and acute myocardial infarction treated with thrombolytic agents. J Am Coll Cardiol 1993;21:920-925.
6. Stein B, Weintraub WS, Gebhart SSP, et al. Influence of diabetes mellitus on early and late outcome after percutaneous transluminal coronary angioplasty. Circulation 1995;91:979-989.
7. BARI Trial. Comparison of coronary bypass surgery with angioplasty in patients with multivessel disease. N Eng J Med 1996;335.
8. Engler R, Yellon DM. Sulfonylurea KATP blockade in type II diabetes and preconditioning in cardiovascular disease: time for reconsideration. Circulation 1996;94:2297-2301.

9. Groop L. Sulfonylureas in NIDDM. Diabetes Care 1992;15:737-754.
10. Gerich J. Oral hypoglycemic agents. N Eng J Med 1989;321:1231-1245.
11. Brady PA, Terzic A. The Sulfonylurea Controversy: More questions from the heart. J Am Coll Cardiol 1998;31:950-956.
12. Klimt C, Knatterud GL, Meinert CL , et al. A study of the effects of hypoglycemic agents on vascular complications in patients with adult-onset diabetes. Diabetes 1970;19:747-830.
13. Seltzer H. A summary of criticisms of the findings and conclusions of the University Group Diabetes Program (UGDP). Diabetes 1970;21:976-979.
14. Aquilar-Bryan L, Nichols CG, Wechsler SW, et al. Cloning of the beta-cell high affinity sulfonylurea receptor: a regulator of insulin secretion. Science 1995;268:423-426.
15. Noma A. ATP-regulated K+ channel in cardiac muscle. Nature 1983;305:147-149.
16. Brady PA, Zhang S, Lopez JR, et al. Dual effect of glyburide, an antagonist of KATP channels, on metabolic inhibition-induced Ca2+ loading in cardiomyocytes. Eur J Pharmacol 1996;308:343-349.
17. Nichols C, Lederer WJ. Adenosine triphosphate-sensitive potassium channels in the cardiovascular system. Am J Physiol 1991;261:1675-1686.
18. Gross G. ATP-sensitive potassium channels and myocardial preconditioning. Basic Res Cardiol 1995;90:85-88.
19. Murray C, Jennings RB, Reimer KA. Preconditioning with ischemia: a delay in lethal injury in ischemic myocardium. Circulation 1986;74:1124-1136.
20. Garratt K, Brady PA, Hassinger NL, et al. Sulfonylurea drugs increase early mortality in patients with diabetes mellitus following direct angioplasty for acute myocardial infarction. J. Am Coll. Cardiol 1999;33:119-124.

21. Brady PA, Al-Suwaidi J, Kopecky SL, Terzic A. Sulfonylureas and mortality in diabetic patients with myocardial infarction. Circulation 1998;97:709-710.

22. Klamann A, Sarfert P, Launhardt V, et al. Myocardial infarction in diabetic versus non-diabetic subjects: survival and infarct size following therapy with sulfonylureas. Eur Heart J 2000;21:220-229.

23. Malmberg K, et al. Prospective randomized study of intensive insulin treatment on long-term survival after acute myocardial infarction in patients with diabetes mellitus. BMJ 1997;314:1512-1515.

24. Malmberg K, Ryden L, Efendic S, et al. Randomized trial of insulin-glucose infusion followed by subcutaneous insulin treatment in diabetic patients with acute myocardial infarction (DIGAMI) study: effects on mortality at 1 year. J Am Coll Cardiol 1995;26:57-65.

25. Diaz R, Paolasso EC, Piegas LS, et al. Metabolic modulation of acute myocardial infarction: the ECLA Glucose-insulin-potassium pilot trial. Circulation 1998;98:2227-2234.

26. Fath-Ordoubadi F, Beatt KJ. Glucose-insulin potassium therapy for treatment of acute myocardial infarction: an overview of randomized placebo-controlled trials. Circulation 1997;96:1152-1156.